THE TRUTH ABOUT
DIVORCE

THE TRUTH ABOUT DIVORCE

MARK J. KITTLESON, PH.D.
Southern Illinois University
General Editor

WILLIAM KANE, PH.D.
University of New Mexico
Adviser

RICHELLE RENNEGARBE, PH.D.
McKendree College
Adviser

Barry Youngerman
Principal Author

☑®
Facts On File, Inc.

The Truth About Divorce

Written and developed by BOOK BUILDERS LLC

Facts On File, Inc.
132 West 31st Street
New York NY 10001

Library of Congress Cataloging-in-Publication Data

The truth about divorce / Mark J. Kittleson, general editor; William Kane, adviser; Richelle Rennegarbe, adviser; Barry Youngerman, principal author.
    p. cm.
Includes bibliographical references and index.
ISBN 0-8160-5304-9 (hc : alk. paper)
1. Divorce. 2. Marriage. I. Kittleson, Mark J., 1952– II. Kane, William, 1947– III. Youngerman, Barry.
HQ814.T79 2004
306.89–dc22   2004010236

Facts On File books are available at special discounts when purchased in bulk quantities for businesses, associations, institutions, or sales promotions. Please call our Special Sales Department in New York at (212) 967-8800 or (800) 322-8755.

You can find Facts On File on the World Wide Web at http://www.factsonfile.com

Text design by David Strelecky
Cover design by Cathy Rincon
Illustrations by Jeremy Eagle

Printed in the United States of America

MP Hermitage 10 9 8 7 6 5 4 3 2 1

This book is printed on acid-free paper.

CONTENTS

LIST OF ILLUSTRATIONS

PREFACE

In developing this series, The Truth About, we have taken time to review some of the most pressing problems facing our youth today. Issues such as alcohol and drug abuse, depression, family problems, sexual activity, and eating disorders are at the top of a list of growing concerns. It is the intent of these books to provide vital facts while also dispelling myths about these terribly important and all-too-common situations. These are authoritative resources that kids can turn to in order to get an accurate answer to a specific question or to research the history of a problem, giving them access to the most current related data available. It is also a reference for parents, teachers, counselors, and others who work with youth and require detailed information.

Let's take a brief look at the issues associated with each of those topics. Alcohol and drug use and abuse continue to be a national concern. Today's young people often use drugs to avoid the extraordinary pressures of today. In doing so they are losing their ability to learn how to cope effectively. Without the internal resources to cope with pressure, adolescents turn increasingly back to addictive behaviors. As a result, the problems and solutions are interrelated. Also, the speed with which the family structure is changing often leaves kids with no outlet for stress and no access to support mechanisms.

In addition, a world of youth faces the toughest years of their lives, dealing with the strong physiological urges that accompany sexual desire. Only when young people are presented the facts honestly, without indoctrination, are they likely to connect risk taking with certain behaviors. This reference set relies on knowledge as the most important tool in research and education.

Finally, one of the most puzzling issues of our times is that of eating disorders. Paradoxically, while our youth are obsessed with thinness and beauty, and go to extremes to try to meet perceived societal expectations, they are also increasingly plagued by obesity. Here too separating the facts from fiction is an important tool in research and learning.

As much as possible, The Truth About presents the facts through honest discussions and reports of the most up-to-date research. Knowing the facts associated with health-related questions and problems will help young people make informed decisions in school and throughout life.

Mark J. Kittleson, Ph.D.
General Editor

HOW TO
USE THIS BOOK

NOTE TO STUDENTS

Knowledge is power. By possessing knowledge you have the ability to make decisions, ask follow-up questions, and know where to go to obtain more information. In the world of health, that is power! That is the purpose of this book—to provide you the power you need to obtain unbiased, accurate information and *The Truth About Divorce*.

Topics in each volume of The Truth About are arranged in alphabetical order, from A to Z. Each of these entries defines its topic and explains in detail the particular issue. At the end of most entries are cross-references to related topics. A list of all topics by letter can be found in the table of contents or at the back of the book in the index.

How have these books been compiled? First, the publisher worked with me to identify some of the country's leading authorities on key issues in health education. These individuals were asked to identify some of the major concerns that young people have about such topics. The writers read the literature, spoke with health experts, and incorporated their own life and professional experiences to pull together the most up-to-date information on health issues, particularly those of interest to adolescents and of concern in Healthy People 2010.

Throughout the alphabetical entries, the reader will find sidebars that separate Fact from Fiction. There are Question-and-Answer boxes that attempt to address the most common questions that youth ask about sensitive topics. In addition, readers will find a special feature called "Teens Speak"—case studies of teens with personal stories related to the topic in hand.

This may be one of the most important books you will ever read. Please share it with your friends, families, teachers, and classmates. Remember, you possess the power to control your future. One way to affect your course is through the acquisition of knowledge. Good luck and keep healthy.

NOTE TO LIBRARIANS

This book, along with the rest of the series The Truth About, serves as a wonderful resource for young researchers. It contains a variety of facts, case studies, and further readings that the reader can use to help answer questions, formulate new questions, or determine where to go to find more information. Even though the topics may be considered delicate by some, don't be afraid to ask patrons if they have questions. Feel free to direct them to the appropriate sources, but do not press them if you encounter reluctance. The best we can do as educators is to let young people know that we are there when they need us.

Mark J. Kittleson, Ph.D.
General Editor

DIVORCE
AND SOCIETY

It's the oldest story in the world. Girl meets boy, girl loves boy, girl marries boy, and they live happily ever after. What's wrong with that picture? Nothing, if you ask most people. The old-fashioned ideals, with a few modern updates, are still important.

According to a study of 273 typical college students reported in the *Journal of Divorce and Remarriage* in 2001, even students who come from families with multiple divorces expect to get married eventually. They also don't expect to get divorced; they rate their chances of getting a divorce at only around two on a scale of one to five, even if their parents have divorced more than once.

Life, however, does not always work out so neatly. These days the hard facts are inescapable. A large percentage of those who get married never make it to the "happily ever after" stage. Millions of marriages in the United States end in divorce (the legal termination of a marriage). The country has seen a high rate of divorce since the 1970s. The **refined divorce rate** (number of divorces per 1,000 married women) seems to have declined since 1980 (from 22.6 that year to 18.9 in 2000), but it is still very high by historical standards (for example, it was 9.2 in 1960). In any case, each divorce leaves an impact on people's lives that can last for years.

Some people realize soon after their wedding that they made a mistake. They are the lucky ones; they can split up without causing too much damage to themselves or others and get on with their separate lives. Most marriages last longer. First marriages that end in divorce last on average about seven and a half years, according to a U.S. Census Bureau report in 1996. By that time, many divorcing couples have children, and life becomes complicated for everyone concerned.

HOW WE GOT WHERE WE ARE

Today's patterns of marriage and divorce are very different from the customs that prevailed in the United States up until around 1970. For generations most married people, whether they were happily married or miserable, assumed they would remain married "till death do us part," as many wedding vows put it.

Divorce laws were also based on that assumption. Even if a husband and wife decided that they could no longer live together, most American states refused to grant them a divorce. Generally, one of them had to sue the other for divorce on grounds such as physical abuse (any act causing physical harm), mental cruelty (such as verbal insults), or adultery (sex with someone other than one's spouse). Those seeking divorce had to prove their case using lawyers, psychological experts, and private investigators.

If someone felt unhappy or unfulfilled in a marriage, too bad; neither society nor the courts considered that a valid reason to get divorced. Finding a new partner more to one's liking was not considered an acceptable reason to end a marriage.

If there were children at home, the law wanted spouses to stay together for the sake of the next generation, and for what was believed to be the good of society. Most people in those days believed that a stable society rested on a foundation of stable families. They feared that a large population of divorced men and women would threaten other families and set a bad example for children.

Lawmakers believed they were protecting women and children by making divorce difficult. In nearly all divorces up until the 1970s, the courts gave the wife sole custody of the children. However, women had fewer opportunities to earn a good salary in those days, so divorced wives and children often suffered financially. Better to keep the family together, people believed, so all money would be available for all family members.

By the 1960s, more and more people began to feel that this legal situation had trapped too many people in bad marriages. They argued that in many cases even the children would be better off if marriages were dissolved.

Marriage, many people believed, is a partnership that should be based on love and mutual respect, not economic need. Others believed, in the spirit of the times, that the personal fulfillment of each parent was just as important as his or her social responsibility.

Whatever the reason, a wave of divorce reform swept the country in the late 1960s and 1970s. Within a few years, divorce became a practical option for married couples in most states. Many of them took advantage of the opportunity. In fact, the worst fears of some conservative critics seemed to be confirmed, as millions of families broke apart and a large proportion of children suddenly found themselves in divorced families.

On the other hand, society did not collapse. The majority of the children in divorced families survived, and many even thrived. Researchers still disagree about the net impact of divorce reforms on society, but few political, religious, or social groups in the United States support a complete return to the old ways. Instead, they are trying to find ways to strengthen marriage so that fewer people are driven to divorce. Some have suggested changes that may make the process of divorce less disruptive and harmful when it does become unavoidable. A small but persistent group of people wants to make divorce more difficult to obtain.

If you are a typical teenager, you probably have close friends or relatives who have gone through a divorce. You yourself may be living with a divorced parent, or you may be part of a "blended" family, with a stepparent and one or more stepsiblings, half sisters, and half brothers. If so, you are familiar with some of the special problems, challenges, and opportunities that confront such families, before, during, and after the divorce.

Kids often have difficulty adjusting to divorce and remarriage. Years may go by before things are back on an even keel, and even that slow progress requires a lot of work by parents and children. The entries in this book may provide some help in dealing with these issues.

WHAT ARE THE FACTS AND ISSUES?

In a few years' time, you may be considering marriage. If you do, what is the chance that the marriage will last? Of course, it depends mostly on you and your future spouse, yet nobody lives in a vacuum. Like other people, you may be influenced by the social world around you. Will society help you to maintain your marriage?

With all the changes of recent decades, where do couples stand today? Roughly half of American marriages in the last few decades have ended in divorce or separation (an agreement by a married couple to live apart without getting divorced). Are marriages becoming weaker, or are people just leaving bad marriages and eventually forming new, stronger ones? Also, how many couples do not even bother to get married, choosing to live together instead?

Reliable, detailed, updated answers to these questions are not always available, for a number of reasons:

- States usually report on the number of marriage licenses they issue (permits for two people to get married); the number of actual marriages is probably a bit lower.

- Marriage and divorce fall under state laws and are controlled by state governments. The states do not all collect and report information the same way.

- Many married people go through **trial separation** or a period of time in which the couple lives apart. Should these couples be counted among the divorced or not?

- Many people live together outside of marriage, often with children present. When these couples separate, should they be included in the divorce statistics? So far, the government agencies that collect divorce statistics have not included this population.

- Most statistics are based on government surveys that ask people what their status is. People don't always tell the truth.

Even the statistics that are available can sometimes be misleading. For example:

- Everyone is familiar with the statement that "about half of all marriages end in divorce," yet at any one time, there are far more married people than divorced adults in the U.S. How can that be? Most divorced people remarry. Although many second and third marriages end in divorce, hope springs eternal and most divorced people try again. Eventually, like a game of musical chairs, fewer and fewer remain in the pool of unmarried divorced people.

- As stated above, some people are married and divorced two, three, or four times, while many others marry only once and stay that way. Is it really meaningful to *average* all these people together?

■ Teenage marriages, which have a high failure rate, have become less common in recent years. If there are fewer divorces today, does that mean that today's marriages are better or just that fewer teenage divorces are pulling down the average?

■ At the other end of the age spectrum, men and women live longer today. Older people are less likely to get divorced; maybe the higher proportion of old people in the United States is keeping the divorce rate down.

■ This year's divorces reflect the marriages of the recent and distant past. One can't really tell what will happen to *this year's* marriages, since circumstances and expectations keep changing.

Divorce numbers

Despite the challenges in getting accurate data, certain types of information are worth reporting:

1. **The total number of marriages and divorces.** The U.S. Bureau of the Census collects numbers from the various states. Their most recent full-year totals from all 50 states are for 1998. They show 2,244,000 marriages and 1,135,000 divorces. Both numbers were down a few percentage points from 1997.

The last year with fewer than one million divorces was 1974, when there were 977,000. In 1940, only 264,000 divorces took place—but the total population was smaller too.

2. **Gross divorce rate.** In order to compare figures from different time periods, researchers often use the gross divorce rate, which is the number of divorces for every 1,000 people. The figure in 1940 was 2.0; in other words, for every 1,000 people of all ages, 2.0 got a divorce. By 1974, the rate had more than doubled, to 4.6.

In 1979, and again in 1981, the gross divorce rate reached a historic high of 5.3, but it has been slowly declining since 1982. By 1998 it was down to 4.2, and in 2002 it dropped to 3.9, the lowest rate in 30 years, according to preliminary figures from the National Center for Health Statistics (NCHS).

3. **Refined divorce rate.** The most useful figure for comparing different times and places is the refined divorce rate, the number of divorces per 1,000 married women over 15 years of age. In 1940, only

8.8 out of every 1,000 married women went through a divorce. By 1974, the number had shot up to 19.3, according to the NCHS.

The refined divorce rate peaked in 1979 at 22.8; that means that more than one out of every 50 marriages ended in divorce that year. Then the trend began to change; by 2000 the rate was down to 18.9. In other words, the divorce rate more than doubled in the 30 years following 1940, but has fallen about 17 percent in the 20 years since then.

4. Marital status. The Bureau of the Census reported in June 2001 that as of the previous year, 56.1 percent of all men 15 years and older were married, 10.1 percent were divorced, 31.3 percent had never been married, and 2.5 percent were widowed. For women, the figures were 52.3 percent married, 12.6 percent divorced, 25.1 percent never married, and 10 percent widowed.

Clearly, the number of currently married people is still far greater than the number of currently divorced people, but the difference is not as great as in the past: In 1970, 65.4 percent of men were married and 3.5 percent divorced; the comparable figures for women were 59.7 and 5.7.

One of the reasons for the decline in the currently married percentage was a large number of unmarried couples living together. The 2000 census counted 56.5 million married couples and 3.8 million unmarried couples of the opposite sex living together. Some 41 percent of the unmarried couples had at least one child under 18 living with them, compared with 46 percent of married couples.

5. **Children in divorced families.** In 2003 the U.S. Census Bureau estimated that as of March 2002, nearly 50 million children under 18 years old (70 percent of the total) were living in a two-parent household. Of the rest, almost 7 million were living with a divorced parent and 3 million more were living with a parent who was separated from his or her spouse. Together, the two groups comprise about 13.5 percent of all children. Another 8 million youngsters, or 11 percent, were living with a parent who was never married. Fewer than 3 million children (4 percent) were living in a home with no parents present (usually with grandparents or other relatives). Finally, about 850,000 (1.1 percent) were living with a widowed parent.

In 2001, the Census Bureau reported that in 1996, 5.2 million children were living with one biological parent and one stepparent or adopted parent.

6. **Duration of marriage before divorce.** The NCHS reported in 2001 that according to a survey of more than 10,000 women, one in

five first marriages ended within five years, and one in three ended within ten years. By 15 years, about 43 percent of these marriages had ended.

The report notes that the older a woman is when she first marries, the longer her marriage lasts. For example, 59 percent of marriages with a bride under 18 ended in divorce within 15 years, compared to only 36 percent of marriages with a bride 20 or over. Younger divorced women are also more likely to remarry—81 percent of those divorced before age 25 remarry within ten years, compared with 68 percent of those divorced at 25 years or over.

Who is affected?

Everyone is affected by divorce. Every state, region, and ethnic group reports similar long-term trends. In July 2002 the National Center for Health Statistics issued a major report entitled "Cohabitation, Marriage, Divorce and Remarriage in the United States." It confirmed that the trends of the last several decades—more divorce, separation, unmarried couples, and unmarried parents—had impacted whites, blacks, Latinos, Asians, and Native Americans.

A U.S. Census report on crude divorce rates in 2001 showed that nearly every state reported a range of about three to six divorces per 1,000 population. Only three states saw an increased rate compared with 1990, while 43 states showed declines (four states didn't report).

The issues

Certain issues and problems are common to most marriages and divorces. Some of the questions are outlined here; they are all treated in greater detail in the entries.

Is there a recipe for a good marriage? Probably the most important factor in making a marriage work is choosing the right partner. Some of the qualities that first attract a person to a potential mate, such as looks and charm, may not be that important in building a happy and long-lasting marriage. Reliability, flexibility, and communications skills are usually more important guarantees of success.

Timing is the next major factor. More than anything, that means waiting. Teenage marriages do not have a great track record. If the goal is to avoid divorce, the best course is for a couple to wait until they have at least some idea of their aims in life, such as the relative importance of career, children, and community.

Apart from these basic guidelines, there is no formula for marital success other than thoughtfulness, loyalty, and the willingness to compromise. And, a large measure of good luck.

Can a troubled marriage be saved? Very often it can, especially if the partners feel there is enough worth preserving, such as raising children together or participating in common activities. It helps if partners acknowledge one another's complaints. Sometimes counseling or couples therapy can help in the process.

Should a couple in an unhappy marriage stay together for the sake of their children? That's the million-dollar question. No one should stay in an abusive marriage; and few people would advise a couple who is a little bored to choose divorce as their first option. The cases in the middle pose the real dilemma: couples who are tired of bickering over every decision or who find that their values and goals are no longer in sync. Would they or their children be better off if they divorced?

Marriage researcher and counselor Judith Wallerstein suggests in her book *The Unexpected Legacy of Divorce* that it is a "myth" that children of unhappy parents are themselves unhappy and need to be rescued by divorce. She also reminds couples that divorce does not necessarily end the conflict. "In our study," she writes, "a third of the [divorced] couples were fighting at the same pitch ten years after their divorce was final." She also notes that the children of unhappy couples in the still-married group seemed to have weathered their family's problems better than children of divorce. Wallerstein advises parents to at least consider "staying together for the sake of the kids."

Researcher E. Mavis Hetherington has a somewhat more positive view of divorce. Like Wallerstein, she has worked on large, long-range studies of divorced parents and their children. In her 2002 book, *For Better or For Worse*, she writes that "much current writing on divorce has exaggerated its negative benefits. I have seen it provide many women and girls, in particular, with a remarkable opportunity for life-transforming personal growth."

What is the recipe for a "good divorce"? In many ways, a divorced family is still a family. Sometimes it can even be a happy family, or at least one that functions well and satisfies the changing needs of its members.

The same qualities that make for a good marriage can make divorce easier and its aftermath more tolerable. Parents need to control their emotions and learn to compromise with their former spouse. They should try to understand what their children are going through, and help them maintain their normal lives as much as possible.

Children need to accept that their school and social lives may be somewhat disrupted and that they may have less money in their pockets. Older children should try to be tolerant of their parents as the family adjusts to the many practical and emotional difficulties that accompany a divorce.

What are the best custody arrangements? If possible, both parents should remain involved in their children's lives. How that works out in each individual case depends on many different variables. The solution that makes sense at the time of the divorce may no longer be the best solution three or five years later, so parents and children should all expect their schedules to change with time.

How much child support should each divorced parent provide? As much as he or she can afford. Children should not have to pay the price of their parents' mistakes. Each parent should contribute to the best of his or her ability to help pay for nonroutine items like school tuition, clothing, and extracurricular activities. Beyond the age of 18, when most custody agreements expire, each parent has to consult his or her conscience and wallet in deciding how much to help with college tuition and other expenses.

Can a stepfamily be a successful family? Many children come to love and respect their stepparents. However, their biological parents will hold a special place in their hearts and loyalties as long as they remain in the picture.

Stepkids often feel jealous of their stepparents, stepbrothers and sisters, and half siblings. Those who are able to see the other person's point of view may overcome that jealousy. In the best case, kids can wind up with more than two parents and turn a difficult situation into an opportunity for a richer life.

Should stepparents try to discipline their stepkids? Most experts say stepparents, especially new ones, should let the biological parent take the primary role in discipline. Stepparents should not attempt to take the place of the kids' biological parent.

Are children who grow up in a divorced family troubled and unhappy? Many are, but the majority are not. Divorce is a difficult burden to place on children. Sometimes they learn the wrong lessons— like never to trust another person. In many other cases, they learn to be stronger and more independent as a result of the experience.

What can kids do to make life a little easier in divorced families? They should try to remember that parents—and stepparents—are only human and are probably doing the best they can. Kids should not have to sacrifice their own needs, but they will usually be better off if they meet their parents halfway.

Can children from divorced families build successful relationships and marriages when they grow up? Most long-term studies have found that there are slight differences between children of divorce and other children in their ability to build successful marriages. The differences may be disappearing, as divorce becomes more commonplace. The bottom line is that once children grow up, they must take responsibility for their own happiness, however good or bad their parents' marriage may have been.

Can nontraditional family structures work? Not much research has been done on nontraditional families, especially as compared with the 100 years of research on marriage and divorce. The scant evidence does, however, suggest that couples who do not get married are more likely to break up than those that do, whether or not they have children. On the other hand, if kids find themselves with two responsible, loving parents—married, adopted, biological, foster, or otherwise—they should probably count themselves lucky.

Is marriage as we have known it on the way out? The answer depends on what people consider the essential features of marriage. As in the past, most people still say that raising children together is the most important part of marriage. Many parents have even rediscovered the benefits of having one stay-at-home parent, and that parent is still usually the mother.

One change that has taken hold is that married fathers spend more time with their children than their own fathers did. Another change is that interethnic couples are finding it easier to get married and be accepted by their families. In addition, many same-sex couples are seeking the right to be legally married. Some people consider that a threat to traditional marriage, but the controversy itself demonstrates that Americans still take marriage seriously.

In the 1960s and 1970s divorce laws were liberalized in America, and the divorce rate skyrocketed. Overall, was the change good or bad? It is easy to find pluses and minuses on both sides of the question. Divorce has saved many people from terrible marriages; it has given a second chance to millions, many of whom have used it to build more fulfilled lives.

On the negative side, many children have suffered unhappiness and insecurity for an extended period of time, sometimes stretching into years of turmoil. Parents have also discovered that divorce can add a new layer of insecurity, financial woe, and conflict. In the end, each person's answer depends as much on his or her view of happiness and morality as on the published research.

RISKY BUSINESS CHECKLIST

If your parents are going through a divorce, here are some things you should avoid if you want to make the best of a bad situation:

- Don't blame one parent for the divorce
- Don't tell tales about one parent to the other
- Don't refuse to help a parent do extra chores around the house
- Don't become angry if an allowance is reduced due to the financial hardship of divorce
- Don't misbehave at school, drink or take drugs, or punish yourself in other ways
- Don't be openly hostile to a parent's new friend
- Don't refuse to give a stepparent a chance
- Don't refuse to give a stepbrother or stepsister a chance

Few people are surprised when an "operatic marriage" (one with lots of drama, shouting, and even violence) ends in divorce. But most troubled marriages are not that noisy or obvious. In fact, many married people claim they are totally surprised when their spouse files for divorce. They might not have been so clueless if they had paid attention to the warning signs of a marriage in trouble.

Risk factors: what can't be helped

Most marriages start out with a disadvantage or two. While no one can change the past, individuals may be better able to overcome it when they know what to look for. Here are a few red flags:

- Either partner is divorced.
- Either partner has divorced parents.
- The couple has lived together before marriage.
- Either partner is under 20 years old.

- The couple gets married after knowing each other only a few months or less.
- The two spouses have different religious backgrounds or beliefs.
- The two spouses have different values relating to marriage and family.
- Married life begins under a financial cloud—debts or obligations are greater than likely income.
- One or both partners cannot handle problems or disappointments well.

Risky behavior for married people that can lead to divorce

Whatever strong points a couple has, they may be in trouble if either partner engages in any of the following behaviors:

- Alcoholism or other substance abuse
- Violence or psychological abuse
- Sex with other people, especially ongoing affairs
- Unequal division of labor (including both household chores and work outside the home)
- No effort to develop common interests or activities
- Unemployment (especially among husbands)
- Inadequate sex life (in the opinion of one or both partners)
- Nagging or constant faultfinding
- Negative styles of talking and arguing (insults, blaming, not listening, silence)
- Low commitment level; putting other things first

Risky behavior for parents in divorced families

Even after two people are divorced, the way they behave toward each other may affect their well-being and that of their children. Here are some things people do that make for a "bad divorce":

- Hiding joint financial assets
- Failing to pay spousal or child support

■ Violating custody and visitation agreements repeatedly

■ Moving to another state with the children

■ Criticizing the other parent in front of the children

■ Sending messages to the other parent through the children

■ Bad-mouthing the other spouse to employers or business associates

■ Making it difficult for the children to see the other parent's family

■ Being too affectionate or sexual with new partners in front of the children

■ Failing to coordinate parenting and discipline styles with the other parent

■ Having unrealistic expectations about stepfamilies

■ Reducing or losing contact with the children (noncustodial parent)

It is easy to list the risk factors, but probably not so easy to correct the risky behaviors. No one, especially a child going through a family divorce, can be perfect. But sometimes just trying can help; when you show loved ones that you understand a bit of what they're going through, they may be more willing to listen to your own special needs in return.

A TO Z ENTRIES

■ CHILD SUPPORT, SPOUSAL SUPPORT

Child support is the money paid by one parent to help cover the cost of food, clothing, and other expenses for a child or children with whom he or she does not live. A court orders those payments, as part of a separation or divorce agreement. Spousal support refers to regular payments made by one divorced spouse to the other also as part of a separation or divorce agreement.

Most families face money worries now and then, but they usually face them as a team. Husbands and wives routinely share their paychecks with each other and their children.

When a couple divorces, both spouses have new expenses, including maintaining a separate home and paying substantial lawyers' fees relating to the divorce. Many may not have much money left over for day-to-day expenses for themselves and their children. Furthermore, divorced spouses often mistrust their ex-partners, and may not want to hand over money to a spouse they have no control over.

Typically, the parent who has **physical custody** of the children faces the most money worries. She or he may not be able to hold a full-time job due to the burdens of child care but still has to pay for the children's daily expenses. That's why most divorce settlements have provisions for child support and/or spousal support.

ALIMONY OR SPOUSAL SUPPORT

Before divorce became widespread—up to around 1970—divorced men almost always had to pay **alimony** to their ex-wives, often for the rest of their lives, or at least until their ex-wives remarried. Alimony—from the Latin word *alimonia,* meaning "sustenance"—is another word for spousal support.

In those days, many Americans believed that a husband had the primary financial responsibility for sustaining his wife and children; wives were responsible for keeping house and raising the children. Judges believed that divorce did not free husbands of their responsibilities, especially if they were at fault. Also, most women could not find well-paying jobs, due to discrimination or because they had left the workforce to become housewives.

State standards for alimony varied greatly, as did enforcement. Some ex-husbands were financially unable to pay alimony and child support. Others refused to pay, claiming the system had treated them unfairly. Still others simply moved to another state, in effect putting them beyond the law.

In recent decades, divorce laws and customs have changed so much that most people have stopped using the term *alimony*. Instead, they began to refer to alimony as spousal support. In any case, it is no longer an automatic part of divorce. Some divorce settlements make no mention of spousal support or limit its size and duration.

The shifting role of the sexes is responsible for much of this change. Today's husbands tend to share at least some of the burdens of child care and housekeeping both before and after divorce, while many more wives work outside the home and earn more than what women earned years ago.

Instead of aiming for a monthly payment of spousal support, which can often be late or missed entirely, women today are more likely to seek a better share in the property distribution at the time of divorce. In fact, women have been getting a better deal than in the past, especially in the **equitable distribution** states.

Community property states give each spouse half of the couple's assets upon divorce. In the past, states that have equitable distribution laws divided assets based on whose name appeared on deeds or bank accounts. Very often, only the husband's names appeared on those documents. Today, courts in those states tend to recognize a wife's contribution to her husband's education and business. The judge may grant her a lump sum payment upon divorce to compensate her.

Although spousal support is far from automatic, it is still fairly common, and the ex-husband is usually the one who pays it. Today judges usually limit the duration of these payments; they expect the wives to use the time to become self-sufficient by upgrading their skills and, in some cases, by returning to full-time work. These short-term payments are often called **spousal maintenance**.

As soon as a couple files for divorce, courts may order one spouse to pay the other **temporary support**. These monthly payments continue until the divorce is finalized. If the final settlement provides for spousal support, such payments are called **permanent support**. The term is misleading, since the payments usually last for only a limited period of time—perhaps a few years. In most states, courts reserve lifetime spousal support to a relatively few cases, usually the end of long-term marriages that may leave an older woman with no other means of support. In a few states, "long-term" can mean as little as ten years.

During negotiations, the partner seeking spousal support may agree to a large one-time payment at the time of the divorce rather than insist on monthly payments. That way, she or he never has to worry about late or missing payments. On the other hand, late payments and nonpayment are less common than they used to be, since federal law now requires that states enforce each other's divorce settlements.

Judges must examine the facts of each case when deciding whether to award spousal support and when fixing the appropriate amount. They often consult guidelines provided by state laws. The primary factors are the ability to pay and the need for support. If one spouse makes a good living while the other has few marketable skills—yet must also care for small children—the court almost always orders the former to pay the latter, at least for a period of time. On the other hand, if both spouses have similar earnings and plan to share custody of their child or children, a court may see no need for spousal support. For the purpose of determining need, a judge also may take account of property owned by each party prior to their marriage.

Today, most couples use **no-fault divorce**, in which neither party accuses the other of misconduct. However, if a spouse chooses to file for a fault divorce, courts often penalize that spouse if the partner is not in fact found to be at fault.

Q & A

Question: If one spouse can prove that the other did something wrong, is the innocent party likely to receive more alimony?

Answer: Yes and no. In some states, courts do not try to decide who was at "fault" in deciding whether to award spousal support, or deciding how much. However, according to the American Bar Association, as of 2001 the following 28 states (along with the District of Columbia) still take fault into account in making spousal support decisions:

Alabama	Mississippi	Pennsylvania
Connecticut	Missouri	Rhode Island
Florida	Nevada	South Carolina
Georgia	New Hampshire	South Dakota
Idaho	New Jersey	Texas
Kentucky	New York	Utah
Louisiana	North Carolina	Virginia
Maryland	North Dakota	West Virginia
Massachusetts	Ohio	Wyoming
Michigan		

Other factors that may influence a decision for a spousal support order are length of marriage, age and health status of both parties, and the couple's customary lifestyle while they were married. If any of these factors changes over time, each party can petition the court for a change in spousal support based on the new circumstances. If the payer loses his or her job or the recipient remarries, courts often reduce or eliminate payments; conversely, if the payer comes into a large inheritance, the payee might have a chance of getting increased payments.

A divorced spouse who is the **custodial parent** (the parent who has primary responsibility for the children) often prefers to do without spousal support in exchange for more child support. Spousal support is taxable as income, while child support is not. On the other hand, the paying spouse often prefers it the other way around, since he or she can deduct spousal support from income for tax purposes, while child support is nondeductible.

Fact Or Fiction?

A divorced person cannot list child support or spousal support as part of their regular income in order to qualify for a bank loan.

Fact: Not true. Consumer credit laws require lenders to count child or spousal support payments in deciding whether to extend a loan. Such payments represent a large part of some divorced parents' monthly income. Lenders will want to see court records or bank statements showing regular deposits, just as they would want to see pay stubs or any other proof of income.

CHILD SUPPORT

Child support plays a vital role in most divorces involving children under 18. Every state requires that divorcing parents support their children financially. They must provide not only for the essentials—food, clothing, health care—but also for luxuries including private school and vacation, if that is what the children have been raised to expect. A parent's responsibilities toward his or her children do not end when a couple divorces.

According to a U.S. Bureau of the Census report issued in 2002, 62.2 percent (over 7 million out of 11.5 million) of all custodial mothers (who care for their children most of the time) received child support in 1999 from the children's fathers—or were supposed to receive such support.

These figures include mothers who were never married to their children's father as well as those who were legally married and divorced. The percentage of mothers receiving child support is even higher among those who are legally divorced. Unfortunately, about a quarter of women entitled to child support in 2000 reported that they did not receive payments that year, and only half received all the money they were due.

Courts awarded child support to many custodial fathers as well—39.2 percent of them were supposed to receive payments in 1999. Yet more than a third of custodial fathers who were supposed to get child support received nothing at all and another third received only partial payments.

DID YOU KNOW?

Custodial Parents and Child Support

Characteristic	Number (millions)	Percent
ALL CUSTODIAL PARENTS	13.5	
Awarded child support	7.9	58.7
Of those:		
Actually received any child support	5	73.7
Received full amount of child support	3.1	45.1
CUSTODIAL MOTHERS	11.5	
Awarded child support	7.2	62.2
Of those:		
Actually received any child support	4.6	74.6
Received full amount of child support	2.8	45.9
CUSTODIAL FATHERS	2	
Awarded child support	0.8	39.2
Of those:		
Actually received any child support	0.4	64.9
Received full amount of child support	0.2	37.7

Source: U.S. Census Bureau, Current Population Survey, 2000.

Generally speaking, support is paid to the spouse who has primary custody of the children (the parent who lives with the children most of the time) and therefore is paying most of their day-to-day expenses. Even if the custodial parent is wealthier or earns more money, the noncustodial parent has to provide his or her share of support on a regular basis. Demographer Judith Seltzer, a professor at the University of California, Los Angeles, reported in her 1998 book, *Fathers Under Fire: The Revolution in Child Support Enforcement*, that parents who pay child support are more likely to visit their children and take an active parenting role. Her findings were based in part on a survey of some 1,300 divorced parents.

Family court judges sometimes change child support agreements, if there is a major change in financial circumstances—for example, if the paying parent earns more money, or the custodial parent loses his or her job. A change in custody arrangements can also result in a revised payment scale, especially when a child moves from one parent to the other. While judges can modify child support, they almost never completely waive or cancel them.

Typically, support continues until the child reaches the age of 18. Unfortunately, this is just when many kids are planning to go to college.

Psychologist Judith Wallerstein reported in her 2000 book, *The Unexpected Legacy of Divorce,* that 58 percent of the children of divorce in her Virginia Longitudinal Study completed college, compared with 89 percent of the children of intact families in the study. Both groups attended the same high schools and lived in the same middle-class neighborhoods. The reason was clear—only 30 percent of the children of divorce who attended college received steady financial support of any amount from their parents, compared with 90 percent of their friends with married parents.

The laws on child support have undergone substantial changes in recent years. The Family Support Act of 1988 required every state to establish guidelines for child support, review those guidelines every few years, and make sure that the guidelines were being followed in family courts. The guidelines take the costs of health care and health insurance into account as well.

In 1996, Congress passed a major welfare reform law that sought to replace child support payments from the federal government under Aid to Families with Dependent Children (AFDC) with support from the noncustodial parent. Many poor mothers who were divorced or single had come to depend on these payments to support their children.

As part of the new law, Congress set up a national system to track people who were under court order to pay child support. Congress also required that employers report the names of all new hires to the appropriate state agency. If an employee owes child support, the employer must withhold a certain amount from his or her paychecks to make up the shortfall.

Many divorced parents do not live in the same state. Under the Uniform Interstate Family Support Act of 1996 (UIFSA), which every state has adopted, custodial parents are finding it much easier to track their ex-spouses across state lines. Local district attorneys are authorized to help custodial parents who live in other states. They can even seize property if necessary.

As a result of these laws and other government initiatives, child support payments by noncustodial parents nearly doubled from $8 billion in 1992 to $15.5 billion in 1998, according to a White House Report in January 2000. The report said that the National Directory of New Hires had located 2.8 million parents in its first two years of existence.

In the 2000 book, *Child Support: the Next Frontier,* law professors J. Thomas Oldham (University of Houston) and Marygold S. Melli (University of Wisconsin), reported that many of the states had not fully conformed to the Family Support Act of 1988. For example, they have not consistently collected information about how guidelines are implemented with individual families or they have not done surveys about the typical local costs of raising children.

For ex-spouses who were married for a long time or who have children, divorce does not sever the financial ties. Child support and spousal support ensure that these two individuals will be dealing with one another on a regular basis for a period that may range from months to years. They will need a good measure of responsibility, honesty, and mutual respect in their new financial relationship.

See also: Divorce, The Legal Process of; Finances and Divorce

FURTHER READING

Blum, Stephanie I., and Marc Robinson. *Divorce and Finances: Know Your Rights Clearly and Quickly.* New York: Dorling Kindersley, 2000.
Oldham, J. Thomas, and Marygod S. Melli, eds. *Child Support: The Next Frontier.* Ann Arbor, MI: University of Michigan Press, 2000.
Strauss, Steven D. *Divorce and Child Custody.* New York: W.W. Norton & Co., 1998.

■ CHILDREN, PSYCHOLOGICAL EFFECTS OF DIVORCE ON

The emotional impact that a divorce has on children. How does it feel for toddlers, young children, or teenagers when their mom and dad get divorced? Every child is different and every divorce is different, but most people seem to be emotionally affected.

First of all, divorce is never easy. Even when kids are used to their parents fighting, insulting, or ignoring each other, the actual fact of divorce usually has a negative emotional impact. Many children experience feelings of anxiety (fear), depression, guilt, anger, and loneliness; they may be weighed down with grief, as if someone they love has died. Their behavior may change as well. Some respond by getting into trouble in school or with friends. Others find themselves taking on new roles with their siblings and even their parents that may or may not be good for kids their age.

Fortunately, children at any age are usually able to bounce back to a large degree, especially if the family members succeed in building stable new lives. Even so, the first few years of adjustment can be painful. During that period, kids need to know that others have gone through the same problems they are experiencing.

Fact Or Fiction?

As long as parents avoid obvious conflict, their divorce will not cause psychological problems for their kids.

Fact: Not true. Even though high level of conflict between parents (whether or not they divorce) can be unhealthy for kids' emotional life, a 1998 study in the journal *Child and Adolescent Psychiatric Clinics of North America* found that children of any age have great difficulty adjusting to a divorce when it breaks up a low-conflict marriage. For those kids, divorce comes as a shock. At the other extreme, some children seem to benefit from the end of a high-conflict marriage, as long as the divorce itself is quickly resolved.

CONCERN FOR PARENTS

Most children take their parents for granted, and most parents don't really mind this. Under normal circumstances, most kids don't think of their parents as vulnerable people who can be hurt, sad, or fearful. Worrying about a parent should not be a kid's job.

Divorce is not a normal circumstance, and many children begin to look at their parents in a different light during and after a divorce. What they see can be disturbing.

Instead of seeming like a superwoman, mom may look physically and emotionally exhausted, almost helpless in the face of her problems. Dad may seem hurt, angry, or confused, and the kids might fear that he is not able to manage by himself. They may see one or both parents crying or hear them worrying openly about the future. It's hard to feel secure when the people you have always relied on no longer seem like towers of strength.

Kids are usually angry with both parents during a divorce. At the same time, some of them may feel sorry for one or both parents, and may want to do *something* to help out. Unfortunately, children cannot do much, apart from being as understanding and supportive as they can be with each parent. Their parents must solve their own problems.

Naturally, most kids don't want to do anything to add to their parents' pain. They may try to make an extra effort to please them by doing chores or working harder in school. There's nothing wrong with doing so, as long as kids don't expect their efforts to turn their parents' divorce around. Parents are always happy with higher grades, but grades do not ease the pain of divorce.

Nor is it healthy for kids to put aside their own needs and priorities in order to help their parents. Most parents will get through this phase. When they do, they won't want to see that their children have given up their social life, or after-school athletics, or any other activity as a result of the divorce.

Children of divorce may also hurt themselves by failing to be honest about their own needs and preferences. For example, if they want to spend more time with one parent, they may be afraid to tell the other one, not wanting to hurt him or her or make them jealous. Honesty is usually the best policy with divorce, as with other situations.

Finally, divorce may lead some kids to overly deidealize their parents. **Deidealization** is a normal, healthy process in which teenagers learn that their parents are normal people with faults and weaknesses. Like any process, it can be dangerous if it goes too far. Some kids are excessively critical of one or both of their divorcing parents, which is usually unfair to the parents and doesn't help the kids feel good about themselves.

Q & A

Question: Does counseling help kids whose parents are getting divorced?

Answer: Absolutely. In October 2002, the National Institutes of Health reported the results of a study of more than 200 families where parents divorced when the children were 9–12 years old. The children were randomly assigned to different programs, including a "skills training program" that involved counseling sessions with their mothers; the study lasted for six years.

Emotional problems were actually halved for those who participated in the intensive program, as compared with those who were not assigned to the program. Participants also showed significant reductions in behavior problems, drug and alcohol use, and sexual promiscuity.

CHILD AS CARETAKER OR CONFIDANT

Sometimes after a divorce parents find they can barely keep up with all of the new demands on their time. Stay-at-home or part-time working mothers may find they now need to work full time. Some attend night school to improve their skills. Others may begin dating. Most feel overwhelmed emotionally and not able to fulfill all of their responsibilities.

Everyone in the family should respond to a parent's stress by pitching in and helping, but some children go overboard. They may take on much greater roles in keeping house, or try to care for younger kids or for a depressed, sick, or substance-abusing parent at the expense of their own social lives or schoolwork. In a very few instances, children have stayed away from school entirely. These kids may feel guilty about going on with their lives while a parent is suffering. Psychologist Judith Wallerstein wrote in her 2000 book *The Unexpected Legacy of Divorce* that some young children may even think their parents will die if they don't care for them closely.

Of course, these **overburdened children** can be very proud of what they have done. Some may gain a sense of independence and maturity that stays with them as they grow up. In the end, however, they usually come to resent the parent whom they "covered" for. Is it fair for kids to give up their childhood in this way? If this is happening to someone you know, you might advise them to seek guidance from a professional, who might be able to suggest alternatives or compromises that will protect these children.

Some children of divorce find themselves in an even more insidious situation. One or both of their parents may begin to treat them as a **confidant** by sharing intimate feelings and even asking for advice. A child or teenager may be flattered to be thought of as an adult, while also feeling frightened and very uncomfortable. Some psychologists, such as Kenneth M. Adams, warn against what he calls covert or emotional incest, in which a parent turns a child of the opposite sex into a substitute "spouse."

Kids who act as **caretakers** and confidants usually feel stressed. They may become alienated from friends with more typical lives. Also, a child who is treated like an adult at home sometimes feels like an adult in school as well and fails to behave with respect toward teachers.

GUILT AND FEELING RESPONSIBLE
FOR THE DIVORCE

According to psychologist Judith Wallerstein, a child will never believe that a divorce is "no one's fault," as a counselor may claim. Since some kids find it hard to blame a parent, the only one left to blame is themselves.

Most children can think of something they did or did not do that upset their parents at one time or another. But even a troublesome child is not likely to break up a stable marriage. Parents may choose not to share with their children all of the reasons for a divorce, but whatever the true reasons are, a child is almost never able to do anything to change the picture.

TEENS SPEAK

Is It His Fault?

No matter what anyone says, Robert is sure that his parents are getting a divorce all because of him.

"I don't have younger sisters or brothers," he says. "My ma had a problem when I was born, and she got hurt, and so she can't have any more kids. I think that's why they're always fighting over me, because whatever they don't get from me, they're not going to get from anyone."

All the kids at the counseling group at his church tell Robert that a 12-year-old boy is not responsible for his parents' behavior, but he refuses to see it that way.

"I'm not so great in school. I just can't get myself to study like I should. My dad doesn't care, he barely finished high school. But my mother is always crying that she never went to college and I could do it if I tried, because I have what it takes. And then he just yells back at her and takes a walk. Isn't that my fault?"

The truth is that Robert's parents just don't see eye to eye on anything; they can't get along and they have given up trying. Even if Robert got straight A's, there would probably be some other issue to come between them. But Robert won't accept that fact.

"At least if I wasn't such a screwup they wouldn't fight so much, and they could work something out."

Robert's priest still hopes he can convince Robert that he is mistaken. If anything, he might do better in school if he stopped blaming himself for his parents' failings.

GRIEVING

No matter how difficult their parents' marriage was, children usually go through a grieving process when their parents separate, even though they may feel relieved. After all, they may be losing the life they have known since they were born, with all of its joys and troubles. Of course, if both parents are still involved with their children after the divorce, they soon create new routines and traditions that can speed the process of adjusting to the loss of the old familiar life.

ANXIETY AND DEPRESSION

Even kids in intact marriages often face anxieties. Worries and fears seem to be a natural part of growing up. One of the worst fears that kids can have is that their parents may abandon them. Divorce can play into that fear.

Preschool children are especially vulnerable to a fear of abandonment. Experts advise parents to do all they can to reassure youngsters that they will not be left alone. The parents are divorcing each other. Neither one usually wants to divorce the child, but it can seem that way to kids.

Psychologist Judith Wallerstein and *New York Times* science writer Sandra Blakeslee reported in their 1989 book, *Second Chances,* that that the mothers in their study of two-parent families who worked outside the home managed to spend 25 hours a week with their children; after a divorce, these same women spent much more time at work, but an average of only 5.5 hours per week with their kids. Fathers were even more absent, dropping from 20 to two hours per week.

One study of about 100 college students, half from intact families and half from divorced and stepfamilies, found that those from divorced families were more sensitive to stress, as measured by heartbeat and other physical symptoms. The authors, psychologists Aurora Torres, William D. Evans, Sonali Pathak, and Carol Vanci, reported their findings in a 2001 issue of the *Journal of Divorce and Remarriage.*

Depression, an emotional state of ongoing sadness and inactivity, can be difficult to diagnose among adolescents, many of whom go through a variety of temporary disappointments and defeats in the normal course of growing up. Nevertheless, a comprehensive study at Iowa State University, published in the *Journal of Marriage and the Family* in 1999, reported a higher incidence of depression among children going through a parent's divorce.

Occasionally, depression may lead to thoughts of suicide. According to the American Academy of Child and Adolescent Psychiatry (AACAP), in a 1998 fact sheet, "for some teenagers, divorce [or] the formation of a new family with step-parents and step-siblings . . . can be very unsettling and can intensify self-doubts. In some cases, suicide appears to be a 'solution.'" A 1994 study in the journal *Social Science Research* found that "the annual rate of children involved in divorce and the percentage of families with children present that are female-headed is a strong predictor of suicide among young adult and adolescent white males."

Psychologist E. Mavis Hetherington reported in her 2002 book *For Better or For Worse* that many 15-year-olds from divorced and remarried families (one-third of the boys, one-quarter of the girls) seem to be uninterested and uninvolved in family life, a frequent sign of depression. Long-lasting depression can be a debilitating condition. Divorced parents should make sure their children see a therapist or counselor if they see signs of depression in a child.

DID YOU KNOW?

Signs of Depression During Divorce

Persistent sad or irritable mood

Loss of interest in activities once enjoyed

Significant change in weight or appetite

Difficulty sleeping, or sleeping too much

Unusual agitation or retardation

Loss of energy

Feelings of worthlessness or inappropriate guilt

Difficulty concentrating

Recurrent thoughts of death or suicide

The following symptoms *may* be a sign of depression among children or adolescents, especially if they are severe and persistent:

Physical complaints, such as headache, nausea, or sore muscles

Recurrent thoughts of running away from home, or actually running away

Alcohol or substance abuse

Frequent absences from school

Poor performance in school

Frequent outbursts of shouting, crying, or irritability

Lack of interest in friends

Reckless behavior

Difficulty with relationships

Fear of death, or fascination with death

Social isolation

Source: Alabama Law Center.

ANGER AND ACTING OUT

Many studies report that both teens and younger children who are angry at their parents for divorcing may express their feelings through annoying, disruptive, or antisocial behavior at home or in school. For example, in a 1999 article in the *Journal of Child Psychology and Psychiatry*, E. Mavis Hetherington and M. Stanley-Hagan wrote that three of four children showed a deterioration in school performance after their parents' divorce.

Many teens may also engage in self-destructive activities like abusing drugs or taking part in unsafe sex. They know that their parents will be hurt and disappointed by these behaviors, which can be a way of "getting back."

Not every child who acts out is suffering from deep emotional problems. Wallerstein points out in *The Unexpected Legacy of Divorce* that many divorced parents lack the time, energy, and self-confidence to enforce rules and discipline. When kids know their parents aren't keeping an eye on them, they may get the feeling that no one cares what risks they may be taking.

BABIES AND TODDLERS

Most experts agree that babies and toddlers may suffer more than older children from divorce. Although children this young don't understand what divorce is, they do sense a profound change in the amount and quality of attention they receive from both parents.

For example, in a 1996 article published by the National Network for Child Care, psychologist Lesia Oesterreich of Iowa State University reports a list of symptoms that babies and toddlers often exhibit after their parents separate. Babies may show changes in eating, sleeping, and bowel movements. Some may become fretful or anxious. Toddlers often are clingy and won't let a parent out of sight. They may have temper tantrums and revert to babyish behavior that they have already outgrown.

Oesterreich advises parents in this situation to make every effort to maintain as many reassuring daily routines as possible. The **noncustodial parent** (usually the father in these cases) should spend as much time with his child as he did before. If the father is not available, parents should try to enlist a grandfather or other adult male.

Young children have some advantages that older kids may lack. Their mothers tend to be young and are more likely to remarry. Younger kids also do not have to deal with the difficult emotional demands that teenagers face when struggling with the effects of divorce.

NEW STRENGTH FOR KIDS

Although living through a divorce can be hard, in some ways it can be good for one's "character." According to a 1995 article in the journal

Pediatrics in Review, written by psychologists Robert E. Emery and M.J. Coiro, research data consistently shows that children from divorced families tend to be more mature, independent, and resourceful. They are also less likely to be limited by gender stereotypes. In other words, many may become more willing and able to assume the responsibilities usually placed on the opposite sex, such as child care (for boys) and yard work (for girls).

Children may sometimes develop stronger ties with their siblings as a result of divorce. Sociologist Jenifer Kunz, after a meta-analysis of 53 studies of children of divorce, reported in the *Journal of Divorce and Remarriage* in 2001 that "children from divorced homes had more positive sibling relationships than children from intact homes." Such children may have to rely on each other more, and they share many intense experiences, including traveling between parents and dealing with stepfamilies.

Some recent studies indicate that differences have begun to shrink between children from divorced families and intact families. Divorce has become so common that many children may no longer feel the shame and guilt that their counterparts experienced years ago. Also, they can turn to friends who have gone through the same process for advice and moral support.

Whether or not children of divorce suffer long-term emotional effects, it is definitely true that parental divorce is a frightening and difficult experience. Any child placed in that situation needs all the help he or she can get—from family, friends, and mental health professionals. With such help, most kids can expect to get past the crisis; they may even emerge as stronger, healthier young men and women.

See also: Divorce, Adjusting to the Realities of; Generational Patterns and Adult Children of Divorce

FURTHER READING

Bode, Janet and Stan Mack. *For Better, For Worse: A Guide To Surviving Divorce for Parents and Their Families*. New York: Simon & Schuster, 2001.

Stewart, Gail B. *Teens and Divorce*. San Diego, CA: Lucent Books, 2000.

■ COHABITATION

See: Love and Marriage; Marriage Lifestyles, Alternative; Relationships, Types of

■ COMMUNICATION AND COMPROMISE IN DIVORCED FAMILIES

Communication: the transfer of information or understanding from one person to another, and compromise: the give and take that allows people to settle differences in a way that satisfies all parties as much as possible. Communication and compromise in a family involves honestly sharing feelings, needs, and reactions.

Communication is the key to successful compromises for all families, including those that have experienced a divorce. People—including parents—are not mind readers. If people don't communicate their needs, hopes, and fears, they can hardly blame someone if he or she sometimes hurts their feelings. Even if family members communicate well, if they don't compromise, at least some of them will be unhappy, and the others may suffer too.

ADDRESSING COMMUNICATIONS ISSUES

Communication should begin before the divorce. Experts advise parents to talk to their children as soon as they are sure the marriage is over. They should explain *why* they are seeking a divorce in words that their kids can understand. The more children grasp the reasons for the divorce, the less likely they are to blame themselves or have illusions that their parents might still reconcile.

Parents should also explain their practical plans for the immediate future, so kids don't feel their needs and feelings are being ignored. Once family members begin to communicate, they will be better able to talk about the many challenges to family life that divorce usually brings.

Hard as it is for parents to talk about separation and divorce, their children may find it even harder to respond honestly. Sometimes children just can't talk to their parents about sensitive subjects like divorce. Therapists say they should be given time until they are ready, although keeping feelings bottled up for too long is not a good idea.

The sooner that kids and parents get in the habit of talking honestly to one another, the better off they usually are. Parents do not necessarily agree with everything their children say, but they may be more likely to be accommodating to the needs of children who can communicate.

Kids may find it easier to sort through their feelings if they can talk to a grandparent or other adult relative, a teacher, or a family friend. Then, when they are ready to talk to their parents, they will know what to say. Unfortunately, adults outside the immediate family

---

DID YOU KNOW?

Seven Effective Communication Skills

- Awareness—about what's going on now in you, in me, between us, and around us
- Clear thinking—avoiding vague and emotionally charged terms, and building your vocabulary
- Digging down below the surface to identify your real needs, which may not always be what they seem
- Listening empathetically (with your heart)—without agreeing or giving in
- Metatalking—talking about *how* you communicate
- Respectfully asserting—declaring your true needs in a way your listener(s) can *hear*
- Problem solving—using the six skills above to identify and fill your and your family members' needs well enough for now.

Source: Stepfamily Association of America

---

sometimes reduce their contact when a couple is going through a divorce and may not be available to talk to the children. In a 2001 article in the *Journal of the American Board of Family Practice*, psychologist Charles L. Bryner, Jr., reports that only one child in 10 in this situation finds an adult to talk to.

Fortunately, most kids are able to talk freely with people their own age, especially brothers and sisters. Many schools have set up groups for children who are going through a family divorce or whose parents have already divorced. By talking things over in a safe atmosphere, kids can learn from each other how to express their feelings and needs, and how to cope with practical problems.

Men going through a divorce may have more trouble speaking openly with their children than women do. If your father does not initiate conversation, don't assume he's not interested in you. According to Bryner, fathers are often "less emotionally available to the children." They might find it easier to talk to coworkers or even to members of a men's group than to loved ones.

If family members are not ready to talk, they can still communicate their feelings through gestures and deeds. A dad can show that he cares simply by arranging a visit or organizing an outing. E-mail is another way to communicate without having a possibly awkward conversation.

TRYING TO BE FAIR

Every family has its rules, whether openly stated or quietly taken for granted. In most cases, these rules have developed over years of family life. No one sits down and writes a set of family bylaws. As the family situation changes, the rules change—for example, when a new child is born or as kids get older and are able to take on more responsibilities. It may take time until everyone is satisfied that the new rules are fair—for example, that all the kids get a similar allowance or are chauffeured to the same number of activities.

Divorce is one of the largest, most abrupt changes in the life of any family. Typically, less money is available after a divorce. If the children alternate between two homes, more chores need to be done; yet everyone has less time for chores thanks to longer working hours for parents and travel time between homes. Sometimes parents simply cannot be fair. For example, if they gave an older child a generous graduation present before the divorce, they may not be able to do the same for younger children after the breakup.

Kids have a right to complain if they feel they are being treated unfairly. However, they should try to understand that their parents and siblings have needs as well. The more people can look at events from someone else's point of view, the easier it is to come up with fair rules and to occasionally put up with unfair treatment. After all, it probably happens to everyone in the family now and then.

IS COMPROMISE POSSIBLE?

Every argument, including conflicts between ex-spouses, or between parents and their children, has two sides. Sometimes one side wins, sometimes the other, but other choices are often available if people make an effort to find them.

Psychologists suggest that compromise is easier if people can "reframe" the issue in dispute so that it is seen from a different point of view. For example, if a father wants his kids to stay an extra day one week because his own parents are visiting, his ex-wife can agree to the change or stand on her legal rights and refuse. A third alternative would be for both parents to agree to make the schedule more flexible. Perhaps they will agree to let the kids spend an extra day or two with either parent whenever that set of grandparents is in town. With that alternative, everybody wins.

In another example, a divorced mom may feel she can't afford to pay for summer camp. Rather than fight that decision, her older children might offer to work one day each weekend during the school year to help defray the costs. Again, nobody loses, and as an added bonus, everyone feels like they've done their part.

THE ROLE OF THERAPY

When family members can't concentrate because anger, fear, or feelings of rejection are overwhelming, they aren't able to communicate or compromise. Many people find that counseling and therapy can help them deal with such emotions.

People facing a family divorce can choose from various types of therapy. Divorce expert E. Mavis Hetherington reports in her 2002 book, *For Better or For Worse,* that the best results for divorcing parents have come with **behavior modification therapy**, a form of therapy in which people learn to change the way they respond to a situation or problem. Kids, on the other hand, often do well in group therapy, where they meet on a regular basis with other children of divorce, under the supervision of a therapist, to share problems and solutions.

Other forms of therapy include psychoanalysis, in which patients try to uncover unconscious mental processes that may contribute to unpleasant or harmful feelings; play or art therapy, where patients, often children, can come to grips with their feelings through artistic expression, and counseling, in which a therapist or other professional tries to help the patient clarify his or her own feelings and goals.

In October 2002 the *Journal of the American Medical Association* reported positive results from a six-year study of some 200 families in a "skills training" program for divorcing mothers and their children. The program, a form of behavior modification, improved mother-child relations and helped kids overcome "negative thoughts."

Most family members lose in some way during a divorce. However, with communication, compromise, and perhaps help from professionals, they can start to build a new life where one person does not have to lose for the others to feel like winners.

See also: Children, Psychological Effects of Divorce on

■ CUSTODY AND VISITATION

Custody, the legal right to house and care for minor children following a divorce. Visitation refers to the amount of time a parent can spend with divorced children who live primarily with the other parent.

When children learn that their parents are getting a divorce, the first question they are likely to ask is, "Who will I be living with?" In other words, will Mom or Dad have custody of my siblings and me? If they get a definite answer to that question, the next question is, "If I'm going to live with Mom, will I ever see Dad again?" In other words, what kind of visitation rights will the other parent have?

Kids are right to ask. These are the two most important questions surrounding divorce for parents as well as for their children. The answer will impact not only every detail of daily life but also a child's relationship with each parent.

No other set of questions can cause as many disagreements between divorcing parents. Often, the children are the only positive result of an unhappy marriage. Furthermore, couples facing divorce often mistrust each other's motives and judgment; each parent may want to retain as much control over their children's future as possible.

Unfortunately, a lot of time can pass between the decision to get a divorce and the final settlement, including custody arrangements. Kids may often be left in suspense until the divorce papers are signed in court. Even that legal document may not be the final word. Life has a way of upsetting and changing the best-laid plans, especially on such a complicated emotional and practical issue.

Fact Or Fiction?

The divorced parent who spends the least amount of time with his or her kids pays the most in child support.

Fact: Not true. In most states, courts treat custody and child support payments as two separate issues. The basic principle in child support is that parents are expected to contribute financially to their children's needs based on their ability to pay. If the noncustodial parent has a lower income than the custodial parent, he or she may only have to pay a small monthly amount.

On the other hand, since the custodial parent does spend more on routine expenses when their children are with them, the courts will often take those expenses into account in deciding how much each partner must pay in formal "child support." Only California has an explicit formula that reduces the amount of support a parent has to pay in proportion to the number of days the children are scheduled to live at his or her home.

TYPES OF CUSTODY

When someone asks, "Who got custody of the kids?" they usually mean, "Where are the kids living now that their parents are divorced?" The question is more complicated from a legal point of view. The law distinguishes between **physical custody** and **legal custody**. Either type of custody can be sole or joint.

Physical custody

A parent with physical custody decides where the children live and controls their day-to-day lives. In common speech, and even on many Web sites, people often use the word *custody* by itself to mean physical custody.

The parent with physical custody after a divorce may wind up spending almost as much time with the kids as before the divorce, especially if he or she is granted **sole physical custody**. That term is misleading. In divorce law, *sole* really means *primary*. The parent with sole physical custody is called the **custodial parent**. The other parent is known as the **noncustodial parent**, even though he or she may spend a fair amount of time with the kids.

The term *shared physical custody* is sometimes used to refer to a situation in which neither parent is designated the custodian, and living arrangements are relatively open-ended and flexible. Of course, that solution requires a degree of cooperation and trust between parents that is not always possible to achieve.

Split physical custody means that brothers and sisters are separated between their parents, sometimes on the basis of gender. Most judges avoid this option, believing that siblings should be kept together during the trying period after divorce. However, after some time has passed many divorced families move toward split custody as a practical arrangement, no matter what the divorce settlement decreed.

Joint physical custody means that the children spend large amounts of time (usually at least 30 percent) with each parent. They may alternate weeks, or they may split up each week—whatever makes the most sense based on work or school schedules. Joint physical custody works best if the parents live close to each other. Courts do not expect school-age children, even teenagers, to commute weekly over long distances.

The trend toward joint physical custody began in the 1980s. Before then, courts almost always followed the **tender years doctrine**, which made women the sole custodians of children under eight years old. As more mothers worked outside the home and more fathers performed at least some "homemaker" tasks, courts began to award parents joint physical custody.

At about the same time, psychologists and sociologists began paying more attention to the special role fathers play in raising well-adjusted children. According to Frank Mott, a senior research scientist at Ohio State University, many experts now believed that without a father's presence, some boys were more likely to become troublemakers at school, and some girls were more likely to adopt risky sexual behaviors.

In 1979 California passed a law that told courts to grant joint physical custody to divorcing parents with children whenever possible. Many other states followed California's lead. Within 10 years, this previously rare arrangement was impacting about 20 percent of all divorces with children.

Divorce mediator Joan B. Kelly, writing in 2003 for the World Wide Legal Information Association, estimated that fathers got sole physical custody of their kids in about 15 percent of divorces in the 1990s, up from about 10 percent in the 1970s and 1980s. These figures are based on U.S. census data and surveys of actual living arrangements. Individual states do not collect data about custody arrangements in divorce settlements under their jurisdiction.

Information about living arrangements (among divorced as well as unmarried parents) show differences among economic and ethnic groups, although the reasons for this are not always clear. Joint physical custody is more common among more well-to-do families and also among whites as opposed to other ethnic groups.

Joint physical custody usually ensures that both parents remain intimately involved in their kids' futures and have the opportunity to give them the love, attention, and support they need. On the other hand, some kids find the situation confusing, especially if their parents have different styles of discipline and different routines. It can also complicate life, especially if the parents live more than a short distance apart.

DID YOU KNOW?

Single Moms and Dads in the United States

Numbers are in millions of parents.

Characteristic	Single Fathers	Single Mothers
Single parents with own children:		
Under 18	2.04	9.68
Under 12	1.44	7.33
Under 6	0.82	4.12
Under 3	0.51	2.31
Under 1	0.20	0.82
Number of own children under 18		
1 child	1.30	5.24
2 children	0.54	2.94
3 children	0.15	1.01
4 or more children	0.06	0.48
Marital status		
Never married	0.69	4.18
Married, but spouse absent or separated	0.35	1.72
Divorced	0.91	3.39
Widowed	0.09	0.39
Poverty status		
Below poverty level	0.33	3.31
At or above poverty level	1.72	6.38

Source: U.S. Census Bureau, 2000.

In 2002 the *Journal of Family Psychology* published an article by researcher Robert Bauserman that summarized 33 studies of custody arrangements over nearly two decades. Bauserman concluded that "children in joint physical custody are better adjusted, across multiple types of measures, than children in sole (primarily maternal) custody."

According to divorce lawyer Mary Ann Mason in her 1999 book *The Custody Wars*, the evidence is more ambiguous. Some studies show that "joint custody does not work well in high-conflict families." In addition, a 2003 study by researchers Carol George and

Judith Solomon found that babies whose parents have divorced or separated "have difficulty establishing secure attachments to their parents" if they move between their parents' homes.

Some experts believe no one solution to custody arrangements is best. Psychologist and author Judith Wallerstein, in her 2000 book, *The Unexpected Legacy of Divorce*, writes, "Joint custody can work very well or poorly for the child." If divorced parents cooperate with each other and the kids are flexible, it can work well. Wallerstein strongly recommends against joint physical custody when the two homes are so far apart that kids can't play with their usual friends or participate in after-school activities while living with the second parent.

Since the evidence about the relative benefits of sole versus joint physical custody is ambiguous, state lawmakers no longer view joint physical custody as the preferred option. For example, the 1979 California law was changed to make it just one option among many.

A few creative parents invented a new form of joint physical custody that they called birdnesting or nesting. The kids stay in one home while their parents take turns living with them. Birdnesting was popular for a time, but many parents found it too difficult to shift back and forth.

Legal custody

According to lawyer Steven D. Strauss, legal custody is "the right of the parent to make medical, religious, educational, and all other important decisions regarding the children." The parent with legal custody decides what school the kids will attend, whether they attend religious services, and what kind of medical or psychological treatments they may receive.

Courts typically appoint both divorced parents as legal custodians, in the hope that they both remain involved in their kids' lives. However, if the couple has a history of conflict over religious or medical issues, judges may grant sole legal custody to one parent. Of course, when one parent is absent or in some way unfit to be a parent, the remaining parent usually gets sole legal custody.

State lawmakers in recent years have tried to protect the legal rights of noncustodial parents. Such parents are now usually granted equal access to educational and medical information about their children and can make emergency medical decisions while their children are in their care.

VISITATION

Whenever a court awards sole physical custody to one parent, it almost always grants visitation rights to the other parent. In doing so, the court allows the noncustodial parent to visit with his or her children for predetermined amounts of time.

Some divorce settlements call for **reasonable visitation**, leaving it up to the parents to work out a flexible schedule. Often, however, parents follow the advice of mediators and counselors and agree on a **fixed visitation schedule**.

A fixed schedule usually provides for holidays, birthdays, and other unique events. It even specifies the time of day that the kids return home, and which parent is responsible for driving the children to and from each visit, in order to prevent misunderstandings and avoidable conflicts.

Once the divorce settlement is approved, visitation, like custody, is binding for both parents. Even if a parent is behind in spousal or child support payments, the other parent cannot interfere with the visits. A parent who tries to keep his or her kids from visiting or returning to the other spouse is in contempt of court and can be fined or even jailed. Still, judges are usually less strict about enforcing custody provisions than they are about property division and child and spousal support. Minor violations are rarely prosecuted.

Some parents fail to live up to their custody responsibilities. Sometimes a noncustodial parent moves away to take a better job. In other cases, he or she remarries and the children do not get along with the new spouse. At other times, a noncustodial parent may find childcare and discipline too difficult. In any of these instances, children may find that their noncustodial parent misses visits and eventually stops showing up at all. Parents cannot be forced to use the visitation rights granted in a divorce.

When the court believes there is an immediate danger that a noncustodial parent might harm the children through abuse or neglect, it may order **supervised visits**. In that case, a neutral third party, sometimes appointed by the court, is present every time the parent sees his or her children.

Q & A

Question: Do grandparents have visitation rights after a divorce?

Answer: State laws vary, but in most states, courts will allow grandparents to file for visitation rights if their grandchildren's parents are divorced.

Most children who have grandparents nearby know how important they can be, especially at times of stress and confusion. After examining 155 children of divorce, the authors of a study reported in the *Journal of Family Psychology* in September 2002 concluded that "greater closeness to grandparents was associated with fewer adjustment problems."

In fact, many single custodial parents count on practical or financial help from their own parents during the transition period. But sometimes the anger of divorce spills over to the older generation, and parents may try to use their custody rights to keep their in-laws from seeing their kids. Grandparents may then have no other alternative but to seek a court order.

WHO DECIDES, AND HOW?

When it comes time to decide which parent or parents should be awarded custody, and how much visitation a noncustodial parent should get, courts consult a variety of people—parents, lawyers, judges, mediators, counselors, and others. Children, however, are not always consulted, especially children under 14. Even when they are consulted, judges will not always honor their wishes.

Many parents agree on custody and visitation terms on their own, without the help of mediators, lawyers, or judges. Even so, these parents usually are influenced by the decisions of judges in previous cases; such decisions can act as guidelines for reaching a realistic agreement that holds up in court.

When judges order or approve custody terms, they are supposed to be guided by the best interests of each child (his or her future health, happiness, and security). Some of the factors they consider are:

- The parenting abilities of each ex-partner
- Each parent's physical and mental health
- The age and health of the children, and their lifestyles and activities
- The parent who has been the **primary caretaker** of the children (has spent the most time raising them)
- The practical ability of each parent to be present and provide for the necessities of life

- The willingness of each parent to cooperate and encourage their ex-spouse to play a parenting role
- The children's stated desires

Some states have formal lists of criteria such as these, but nearly all states allow for flexibility.

In recent years, groups that advocate to protect the rights of divorced men and women have joined the public debate over custody rules. For example, they have argued about what tasks should be included in deciding which parent has been the primary caretaker.

CHANGES IN CUSTODY OVER TIME

No custody arrangement is perfect. Younger children in particular often miss whichever parent they are not with at the moment. Other kids may find the schedule impractical or may prefer to spend more or less time with one parent. Teenagers may not want to spend much time with either parent; schoolwork, jobs, sports, and socializing may leave little quality time for parent-child bonding, no matter where the children are sleeping every night.

Many divorce settlements now include explicit provisions for changing custody and visitation arrangements over time, as children pass through the stages of childhood and adolescence. When custody changes, child support payments may also need to change. Parents can make these changes voluntarily, and they can also ask the court to update the original divorce agreement to reflect the new arrangements.

TEENS SPEAK

It Just Makes More Sense

Karyn and Troy are two teenagers who live in a small town in West Virginia. They were nine and seven years old when their parents divorced five years ago.

Karyn wasn't surprised when her parents told them what was happening: "Hello, they were fighting all the time."

"It was *not* all the time," Troy insists, but Karyn says, "Stop being a baby." She explained, "Troy still blames Mom because she's the one who wanted the divorce. That's why he wanted to live with Dad."

"As if anyone cared what *I* said."

In the divorce agreement, the judge gave joint custody to both parents. The kids would spend school days with their mother, and weekends and half the summer with their father.

"It was a big pain," Karyn explained. "Dad had to stay at this old house his parents had, like miles and miles away. Anytime I wanted to see my friends over the weekend, I had to beg him to drive me. I'm 14 years old now, I can't sit home and play with dolls. Of course, Junior here got to go fishing all the time."

"The kids are cooler down by Dad's anyway. And the middle school has the best soccer team."

For two years, Karyn and Troy were driven back and forth every Friday and Sunday night. Karyn kept complaining about her social life, and Troy usually didn't want to go back Sunday nights. Finally, last August their parents agreed to change things around for the new school year.

"Now we spend every Sunday together with Mom and her family," Karyn explained. "At night Troy goes back to Dad. I kind of miss Dad, but this summer the three of us are going on a camping trip in the Smokies, so I have that to look forward to."

"And Mom has really mellowed out," Troy added. "She seems to appreciate me better one day a week. It just makes more sense all around."

Any parent who believes that the other parent has become a less capable parent since the settlement was signed can try to have custody modified. Judges are usually unwilling to make changes at the request of one party, unless it is clear that the new circumstances will seriously damage the best interests of the children.

Every divorced family is different. No one can come up with a custody formula that applies equally well to every situation. However, the experience gained in the last few decades, when divorce became so common in the United States, will help guide parents and divorce professionals in the future. With a little bit of good faith all around, most families may be able to develop a workable plan that suits everyone as best as can be expected.

See also: Divorce, The Legal Process of

FURTHER READING

Dimick, Janice M., and Kenneth M. Dimick. *Child Custody: Achieving a Parenting Partnership.* San Jose, CA: Resource Publications, 2002.

Mason, Mary Ann. *The Custody Wars: Why Children are Losing the Legal Battle and What We Can do About It.* New York: Basic Books, 1999.

Roleff, Tamara L., and Mary E. Williams, eds. *Marriage and Divorce: Current Controversies.* San Diego, CA: Greenhaven Press, 1997.

Strauss, Steven D. *Divorce and Child Custody.* New York: W.W. Norton & Co., 1998.

■ DIVORCE, ADJUSTING TO THE REALITIES OF

The strategies children have developed to survive the emotional effects of their parents' divorce.

For some kids, the news that their parents are going to divorce may come out of the blue. For others it may not be a surprise at all. Some parents may even go through a long period of indecision, a "roller coaster" of hopes and disappointments. Sometimes parents do manage to work it out, to put the pieces back together again.

All too often, however, parents go through with the divorce. Their kids may have hoped it wouldn't happen, but it did. Now they must learn to live with it. It isn't easy, but if it happens to you, you won't have to reinvent the wheel. You can benefit from the experience of other kids, who had to face many of the same challenges that are confronting you.

SADNESS AND GRIEVING

After getting over the initial shock and that panicky thought, "What will happen to me?" most kids react to divorce by feeling very sad.

When things go wrong, people tend to feel sorry for themselves. They remember the happy times they shared that may never return in the same way. They think of the sacrifices they may have to make. A teenager will rightly ask, "Isn't my life supposed to be filled with new experiences that *add* to my happiness, not subtract from it?"

Many kids also feel sad for their parents, for the pain and hurt they are probably experiencing. You love your mom and dad, yet sometimes it seems as if all they can do is hurt each other. It can be discouraging to find out that your parents aren't perfect, the way you probably thought they were when you were a little kid.

Counselors and therapists have discovered that most people react to a serious loss by going through certain emotional stages. Psychiatrist Elizabeth Kubler-Ross, in her 1969 book *On Death and Dying,* discerned **five stages of grief** that people usually go through when they are incurably ill or when a loved one has died or is close to death. The stages are denial, anger, bargaining, depression, and acceptance. Other therapists soon adopted her concepts and applied them to other losses including divorce, which can cause people to grieve almost as if a loved one had died. Kids going through their parents' divorce often experience these five stages.

The denial phase ("They're just having one of their fights, they'll get over it") can be a safe first reaction. People often refuse to face the truth if it is too much to handle right away. After a while, though, it is better to face up to the truth, if only to prepare for the problems that are sure to come.

People may say that anger never solved any problem, and perhaps they're right. But who can really blame children for being angry when their parents turn their whole world upside down? The anger stage is a natural reaction. It doesn't help to keep feelings bottled up, but eventually people have to deal with the divorce and it is a lot easier to do so once they have gotten past their anger.

The next stage is bargaining. A kid may try to bargain, reasoning "Maybe there's something I can do that will bring my parents together." Nice try, but divorce is almost never about what the *kids* did or didn't do, so how can *they* fix it? When people finally understand that they can't put things back to the way they were, that's when depression often begins.

Someone who is depressed feels sad all the time, unable to enjoy life, tired without reason, and hopeless. Depressed people may find it hard to perform day-to-day tasks at home, work, or school. Sometimes depressed people even think of suicide.

The final stage is acceptance, when people come to understand that what was lost cannot be regained, and learn to live with the new situation. To reach this stage, kids often find it helpful to talk to a neutral adult, someone who is not personally involved, as a relative might be. A good idea may be to talk to a guidance counselor or school psychologist.

If you ever find yourself in this situation, ask your mom or dad or a teacher you like to make the appointment if you're shy. The counselor may be able to direct you to support groups in your community, where you can talk to other kids who are experiencing similar problems. Other resources might include a coach, scoutmaster, religious leader, or a neighbor.

MAINTAINING IDENTITY

So many things change when a family goes through a divorce, but one thing doesn't change—you are still you. Your mom may no longer be a wife, and your dad not a husband, but you are still the same person you were before. Psychologists say that the best thing you can do for yourself is to stay that same person no matter what you have gone through.

You may have to make an effort to stay the same. First of all, try to keep in touch with relatives—grandparents or aunts and uncles. You are still their grandchild or relative, and they are probably anxious to stay close to you too. In the past, your parents made the arrangements to get together; now, you may have to take the initiative.

It may be a bit uncomfortable at first. For example, it wouldn't be surprising if grandparents choose sides, maybe by sympathizing with their own child instead of their former son- or daughter-in-law. Try to find fun activities to do together, or other topics to talk about, and you can probably avoid negativity and strengthen these important family ties.

Let your parents know of your interest. They may not always find it easy to deal with their former parents-in-law, but they should understand that it is in your best interest to stay on good terms with everyone.

Next, make sure to keep a strong profile with your friends and at school. If your parents have shared custody, you may be spending a lot of time traveling, or passing time in a new neighborhood. Try not to let old friendships suffer. Your friends are an important part of who *you* are. Just hanging out with them, throwing a ball around, or seeing a movie can help you feel like your old self again.

If you have always been active in sports or after-school activities, that should not change now. Try to keep up these activities, even during the difficult transition period. Attend scout meetings or teen programs at your school, place of worship, or community center.

Kids sometimes let their schoolwork suffer when their parents get divorced, perhaps as a way of punishing them. Such childish behavior is self-defeating and can only increase tension and anger among family members.

On the other hand, it may not be to your advantage to go to the other extreme and try to be the second adult in the house. You may have to pitch in a little more, like babysitting for a younger sibling or doing some of the heavy chores, but you have a right to be a kid until you physically grow up.

PARENTS DATING

You may be starting to date, or you may be thinking about it. What if your divorced dad or mom is dating too?

Some kids may think, "They had their chance. Now it's my turn." But remember to be fair. You may want your parents' full attention, but they've been through a lot. If they need to get out a little, shouldn't you cooperate? As much as they love their kids, they probably feel lonely. Adults need some adult company now and then; it can even put them in a better mood.

If you are like most kids, you may feel a little worried. Will the new friend take your place in your parent's heart? Will your parent still have enough time for your needs? If the friend has children of his or her own, does that mean that even more disruptions are in store? Is a whole new "stepfamily" about to take shape?

You have a right to ask these questions, respectfully, and to get honest answers. However, try not to make snap judgments about your parents' dates. If your own friend shows up wearing weird clothing, would you want your parents to jump to conclusions? Remember, this is not your date; it's your mom's or dad's.

TEENS SPEAK

What Goes Around Comes Around—
Waiting Up for Dad

Mark and Karyn are 16-year-old fraternal twins, whose parents got divorced about two years ago. The kids really took it hard. They still don't like it, but sometimes weird things happen that make them laugh, and then it somehow gets a little easier.

The twins get to see their dad every other weekend.

"At first," Mark said, "it was so icky. Uncomfortable. We never spent that much time alone with Dad even before the divorce, so he didn't really know what to do with us."

Karyn interrupted, "It was like he had this book, *50 Things Dads Can Do with Their Kids so They'll Think He's Cool.*" She rolled her eyes. "So when he asked us one Friday in the car if we minded if he went out on a date Saturday night, we were like, 'Please do!'

"He's got all these cool DVD's anyway, so we just camped down in front of the tube," Mark said. "When we finished one, we popped in another. Then it was eleven, then it was midnight. Where's Dad? Sis here started to get real worried."

"Well, he's so strict. I started going out on double dates this year, and would you believe Dad calls Mom every hour to find out if I'm home yet. So I thought, he's so punctual, something awful must have happened."

"We couldn't focus on the TV. Karyn kept going to the window every five minutes; I wanted to call the police."

"Finally he showed up at 12:15," Karyn said. "I marched downstairs and as soon as he opened the door, I shouted out, without thinking, 'You're grounded!' He was so surprised, he dropped his keys right on the floor."

"And then he looked at us, and we looked at him, and we all burst out laughing," Mark said, smiling. "The weekends are a lot better now; we can laugh at dad—no, *with* him."

HOLIDAYS

Most people look forward to holidays as special family times. Everyone makes that extra effort to gather together to celebrate traditions and create new memories. Schools are closed; your brother or sister in college may drive hundreds of miles just to be with you all; your parents take a few extra days off from work to take care of "the really important thing," their family. And you spend the entire week trading visits with relatives and family friends.

What about divorced families? For families who have recently gone through a divorce, holidays can be the most difficult time of all. They remind everybody of the way things used to be, of the way you thought they would always be. Often it seems as if everyone else is having a storybook holiday, while all your time is devoted to dealing with the eternal question: "Which kid will be with which parent on which day?

As time goes on, new traditions will develop and new memories gather. Sometimes you even wind up getting double holidays, birthday parties, and presents.

Even in the first year, children can help. Make sure to remind your parents about birthdays and holidays in advance, so they can make plans. Let them know you need time with your friends as well. Plan to surprise each parent with a thoughtful birthday present or holiday card, which may mean more to them now than ever before. Sometimes when you make the extra effort, the holidays can remind you of what you still have, despite all the troubles you've been through. Isn't that what they're all about?

Divorce may be the most difficult challenge a child has to face. But isn't challenge and change what growing up is all about? In fact, children who adjust successfully to divorce often become more confident than they were before. They may even have a head start as they and their friends embark on their adult lives a few years down the road.

See also: Children, Psychological Effects of Divorce on; Relationships After Divorce, Parents'

FURTHER READING

Krantzler, Mel, Patricia Biondi Krantzler, and William M. Lambers, Jr. *Moving Beyond Your Parents' Divorce.* New York: McGraw-Hill/ Contemporary Books, 2003.

Royko, David. *Voices of Children of Divorce.* New York: Golden Books Adult Publishing Group, 1999.

■ DIVORCE ALTERNATIVES

Options available for couples whose marriage seems to be over but who do not actually divorce.

The marriage is over. Despite every attempt to work things out, a couple agrees that they cannot continue living together as husband and wife. So, they get divorced, right?

Not necessarily. The couple can agree to get a divorce at some future date; a failed marriage can be bearable to a spouse who knows when the suffering is going to end. Also, they can agree to a **trial separation**, which is a legally defined status in which the couple lives apart until they decide what they want to do or until their divorce comes through.

Then again, one of the partners can simply move out without taking any legal action. Nearly five million Americans are married but live apart, according to the U. S. Census of 2000. They live totally separate lives. Some spouses have even lost track of one another.

DELAY DIVORCE

Until the reforms of the 1970s, state laws often required waiting periods before divorce. Even without a designated waiting period, the process often dragged on for months or years, since divorces were always based on fault and often involved a lengthy court fight.

Today, few states still require a waiting period for divorce. One unfortunate result is that families lack the time to think through the consequences of the divorce and make necessary preparations for their new lives. That lack of preparation may lead to greater levels of stress in the crucial period around the time of the divorce.

Some experts believe that at least some marriages would be saved if couples had a waiting period, a chance to cool off. Psychologist Judith Wallerstein suggested in her 2000 book *The Unexpected Legacy of Divorce* that many couples would benefit by consulting an attorney about the financial, legal, and custody implications of divorce *before* they finalize their decision. After examining all of the downsides of divorce, some couples might decide to give their marriage more time, for their own benefit as well as for their children's. For example, if a stay-at-home wife needs to return to school, Wallerstein suggests she do it while still married.

Adding support to these suggestions, a study released by the University of Chicago in July 2002 found that people in unhappy marriages who divorced were no happier five years later than those who were unhappy but stayed married. The conclusions were based on a long-term survey of several hundred people, conducted by the National Survey of Family and Households.

TEENS SPEAK

Confused but Carrying On

Joanne's brothers do not know their parents are planning to get divorced.

"I only found out because I'm always calling my friend Clarissa, and I picked up the phone in the den while my mother was talking. Later on she told me everything. They are going to wait a couple of years, if they can hold out. She was very calm, and I appreciated that she talked to me like a grown-up."

Joanne is almost 15.

"My Dad travels a lot anyway for business, so we sometimes don't see him for a week or two. It hasn't made any difference so far. When he comes home, he takes us to the movies or a ball game, or whatever, and Mother makes an excuse. The whole point is not to put my kid brothers through a divorce, because they're too young—eight and 10. I don't think they know anything yet, they're so wrapped up in their teams anyway."

Is she upset that her parents are planning to divorce, eventually?

"Sometimes I forget all about it. But when I see them together and I know they don't love each other anymore, it's very upsetting. I'm not supposed to tell my friends, so sometimes I feel like I'm going to burst. But it's better that Dad is still here. I would really be scared if he left."

Joanne wants to go away to college. She's hoping her parents stay together until then.

TRIAL SEPARATIONS

Many couples use a trial separation not only to see if a divorce would be right for them but also as a cooling-off period after a difficult time. The word *trial* can sometimes be a misnomer, as some couples use this time as a temporary stopgap if they feel they cannot live together while preparing their divorce.

Some spouses "separate" by moving to a different bedroom or section of the house (or to a vacation home), but in most cases, they change their address. Having a parent move out can be the most traumatic part of the divorce process for kids. After a parent leaves, no one can deny that the family is in crisis.

When a married couple separates, they should formalize the arrangement with a **legal separation** order. Doing so protects either spouse from debts and bills incurred by the other during the separation.

The order can also provide for temporary custody and financial support, while defining each spouse's rights and responsibilities during the separation period.

Divorce attorneys warn that hasty decisions made at the time of separation usually affect the final divorce settlement. For example, if one spouse moves out of the couple's home, judges tend to formalize that arrangement. The division of property in a divorce settlement is also likely to follow the lines established during separation. Furthermore, the future value of pensions is calculated as of the separation date rather than the divorce date.

A legal separation is sometimes called a **bed and board divorce**, or **separate maintenance** in some states. It can actually become a permanent arrangement, which may suit both partners as long as neither wishes to remarry.

In a few cases, separation helps couples decide that they do not really want to divorce, or that the practical difficulties of divorce are not worth the benefits. They may feel that the trial period saved them from a serious mistake.

INFORMAL SEPARATION

Most people ending a marriage prefer the legal protections that accompany a divorce, but not everyone chooses that path. A significant number of married couples separate without formalities. Some of the reasons they take that path include:

- Religious principles: Many older Roman Catholics (and some Baptists) believe that divorce is never acceptable, even if strife or abandonment has physically broken up the home.
- Community traditions: In some communities, the legalities of divorce and remarriage are not considered important as long as the children of the original marriage have a legally recognized father and mother.
- Money and other resources: Nearly every divorce involves financial costs, which can be a significant burden to poor people; in addition, some less-educated people may not have the resources or confidence to seek all the legal protections they deserve.

No one can argue with religious principles or community values. Still, those who lack the resources to follow through with a divorce

DID YOU KNOW?

Percent of Separated Couples Who Divorce Within Three Years

Community characteristic	Percent of separated couples who get divorced
Poverty:	
High poverty rate	72
Intermediate poverty rate	89
Low poverty rate	90
Unemployment:	
High unemployment	72
Moderate unemployment	85
Low unemployment	91
Welfare:	
Many welfare recipients	70
Average welfare recipients	88
Few welfare recipients	92

Source: U.S. Centers for Disease Control and Prevention (CDC), 2002.

would be wise to contact legal aid agencies in their area, especially if they believe they may eventually lose track of their spouse. They may regret their inaction if at some future time they want to remarry, or if they are ever contacted by aggressive debt collectors seeking payment for their spouse's overdue bills.

Separation can be a kind of no-man's land, in which the family is neither intact nor broken up. As such, it can provide at least some comfort for kids facing the difficult prospect of divorce. In some cases, it may lead to a better resolution than anyone had hoped for.

See also: Help for Troubled Marriages

FURTHER READING

Raffel, Lee and Jean Houston. *Should I Stay or Go?* New York: McGraw Hill/Contemporary Books, 1999.

■ DIVORCE IN AMERICA

The statistics and laws on divorce that are specific to the United States. Over the last fifty years, the laws and customs of marriage and divorce have been changing in many countries around the world, not just in the United States. Such changes include the legalization of divorce in predominantly Roman Catholic countries in Europe and South America, the decline of arranged marriages in much of the world, and the rise of greater equality between men and women.

Great changes have come to the United States too. Delayed marriage, **cohabitation** (living together without being married), and divorce have become so common that some social critics even wonder whether marriage is an endangered species. A quick glance into the history of divorce in the nation, however, reveals that change is not a new phenomenon, but has been here since the earliest days.

A DIFFERENT COUNTRY

From the 1600s on, divorce laws were more liberal in colonial North America than they were in England. In particular, the New England Puritans rejected the teachings of the Church of England, which, like the Roman Catholic Church, maintained that marriage is a sacrament that remains valid for life.

Massachusetts and Connecticut colonies took control of divorce from church leaders and gave it to civil authorities, who expanded the legal grounds for divorce. Divorces were still rare—one historian counts only 98 divorces in the colonies between 1639 and 1698—but they were much more common than in England, in proportion to the population. Most divorce suits were brought by men, probably because a woman's property became her husband's as soon as she married.

By the 18th century the numbers of divorces surpassed anything known in Europe. In Connecticut, 390 couples divorced in the 50 years before 1788. In the Southern colonies, on the other hand, divorce was all but unknown, due to the powerful role of the Church of England (and the Roman Catholic Church in Maryland).

Even in New England, the official grounds for divorce were fairly limited. A man could divorce his wife if she committed adultery, but in practice a woman could not divorce her husband for that reason. However, she could divorce her husband on grounds of cruelty, desertion, bigamy, or impotence.

Colonial legislatures, like the British Parliament, had the power to grant individual divorces. They used this power more frequently than

Parliament did. By the 1770s, however, British governors began over-turning divorces in Pennsylvania, New Hampshire, and New Jersey. These actions became one of the grievances that turned many colonists against England.

In some ways, American society was freer and more democratic than European society even in colonial times (apart from the presence of slavery). In England, as in other European countries, divorce was such a complicated and expensive process that only aristocrats or very well-connected individuals could get one, sometimes by a special act of Parliament. In British North America, by contrast, records show that as far back as the 1700s the majority of divorces were granted to poor or middle-class individuals. Many were granted to women, who could not at that time obtain a divorce in England.

THE REVOLUTIONARY ERA

The American Revolution (1775–1781) brought many changes to life in the former colonies, including marriage and divorce. In describing the break with England, many revolutionary writers compared the process to a divorce and remarriage. Some argued that just as the colonists had the right to end their relationship with England and form a new union, individuals should also have the freedom not only to freely enter unions (marriages) but also leave them when there was no longer mutual affection. They believed marriage should be a union of love and support rather than an economic or political arrangement. That idea has stayed with Americans to the present day.

During the revolutionary era, the right to a divorce was considered a way to strengthen families. As Thomas Paine wrote, "We make it our business to oblige the heart we are afraid to lose." In other words, he and others thought people might try harder to please their spouse if they know their spouse could divorce them.

Some writers supported more lenient divorce laws as a way of reducing the high rate of desertion by husbands. Desertion was always fairly common in the colonies. Community ties were weaker, because the population was scattered in widely separated communities under many different colonial jurisdictions. The frontier provided an obvious destination where runaways could find work, "no questions asked." If husbands could get legal divorces, it was argued, they would be less likely to simply abandon their spouses.

Immediately following the American Revolution, several states passed new divorce laws, especially in places where colonial governors had overturned divorce decrees. Even most of the Southern states legitimized divorce by putting it into their statute books. Although the grounds for divorce in the Southern states were more limited than in the North, they did pass laws providing for **legal separation**, which they called bed and board divorce. In a **bed and board divorce**, neither of the ex-partners could remarry, but they were freed from the obligations of marriage. The woman was no longer subject to her husband's control in financial matters.

In both the North and South, the new statutes did not allow for **no-fault divorce** (in which neither party is found guilty of misconduct). In practice, however, judges tended to be lenient and did not require elaborate proof of misdeeds. According to historian Norma Basch, in her book *Framing American Divorce*, county court records from the nineteenth century show that in "the vast majority of cases . . . the defendant failed to appear, a circumstance that contributed to a liberal construction of the statutes."

Yet no one really wanted to see many divorces. Many Americans believed that happy, virtuous families were a guarantee of national virtue and strength. Many people still associated divorce with the perceived immorality of aristocrats. Whenever there was an increase in divorce, social critics warned that the nation was in danger of being corrupted.

EASY DIVORCE SPARKS A REACTION

In the mid-19th century, divorce became even easier for those who lived in the West or had the time and money to travel there. These states were sometimes referred to jokingly as "divorce colonies." State legislators, first in Indiana and later in other states, reduced the residency requirements for those seeking divorce to as little as three months. They hoped that during the waiting period these individuals would spend freely on local hotels and services. Illinois became the destination in the 1880s, followed by several of the Plains states farther west. Nevada retained its reputation as a haven for easy divorces up to the late 1960s.

Q & A

Question: How did Reno become the "divorce capital of America"?

Answer: In the early 20th century, the state of Nevada had some of the most lenient divorce laws in the United States, in keeping with a frontier tradition. In 1906, Laura Corey, wife of the president of U.S.

Steel, moved to Reno, then the state's largest city, and filed for divorce against her husband. The well-publicized and scandalous details put Reno on the map, and dozens of famous and wealthy people followed Corey's example.

In 1927, the legislature lowered the residency requirement to three months; four years later, it slashed it to six weeks. In the following decades, tens of thousands of out-of-staters made the trek to the "divorce capital." Only the liberalization of divorce around the country in the 1970s ended this lucrative "industry" for Reno and Nevada.

The rise of divorce colonies sparked a vigorous national controversy. From 1850 on, newspapers and books were filled with arguments for or against laws that made it easier for couples to divorce. Opponents feared that divorce fed immorality, weakened society, and harmed children. Those who supported liberal divorce laws usually stressed its benefits for women. In fact, the issue of divorce became closely tied to the feminist movement, which was gaining many supporters in the second half of the century.

Through the mid-19th century, men had far greater rights than women in marriage. In most states, a woman's property passed to her husband upon marriage, as did all her earnings during marriage. Men had almost complete legal control over their children as well. Feminist women and their male supporters gradually persuaded lawmakers in state after state to pass laws that gave married women property rights and, some say, rights over their children. They also succeeded in winning a little more acceptance for divorce as a means of freeing women from abusive marriages.

As the United States expanded to the west, new states were added to the union that had been previously settled by people of French and Spanish descent. In French-speaking Louisiana and Spanish-speaking Texas and California, wives kept title to property they brought to their marriages, and both spouses shared ownership of income earned by either spouse during marriage. These preexisting laws continued under the new U.S. territorial and state governments and they eventually influenced the way other states viewed marital property and divorce.

THE MODERN ERA

Throughout the 19th century, divorce rates in the United States were low, compared to those of the next century. By 1900 only three of every 1,000 marriages ended in divorce. By 1920 the rate had soared to 7.7 divorces for every 1,000 marriages. Observers at the time generally attributed the rise to the disruptions and mobility caused by World War I (1914–1919)—in particular the drafting of millions of young men.

Whatever the cause, by the 1920s many ordinary people knew someone who had experienced a divorce, and the social stigma associated with divorce diminished. Public discussions of the topic, in periodicals and lectures, now began to stress the damage to children that divorce might cause. In fact, wide public debate about marriage and divorce helped give legitimacy and win a wide audience for the fields of sociology and psychology.

Most divorces in the early twentieth century were given to women; the most common grounds for divorce was nonsupport—husbands were found to have failed to provide adequately for their wives or children. With the growth of a consumer economy and advertising, courts expected husbands to provide more than basic food and shelter.

THE BIG SHIFT

The divorce rate declined during the Great Depression in the 1930s, as it often does during periods of poverty and unemployment. World War II (1941–1945) and its aftermath brought a temporary spurt in divorces in the 1940s, much like the spurt in the 1920s. By contrast, the 1950s and 1960s saw an increase in marriages, a decline in divorce, and a celebration of stable marriages in movies, television, and popular magazines. That trend, however, did not last. In less than two decades, a combination of legal reform, social and economic change, and new values such as feminism and personal fulfillment dramatically changed both marriage and divorce in the United States.

Fact Or Fiction?

The "great generation" of the World War II era avoided divorce.

Fact: On the contrary, World War II brought a big increase in the divorce rate. In 1946, 610,000 couples got divorced, more than twice as many as in 1940. The divorce rate of 17.9 per 1,000 married women was by far the highest rate in history.

Historians argue about the reasons for these changes, but no one can deny how dramatic they were. According to the United States Census Bureau, the **refined divorce rate** (the number of divorces per 1,000 married women) doubled in just 11 years, from 10.6 in 1965 to 21.1 in 1976. In 1970 all but a small minority of children in the U.S.— 15 percent—lived in two-parent families, about the same percentage as in the 1880s, according to a 1994 Census Bureau report. By 1990, 27 percent of children lived in single-parent families; that number reached 30 percent by 2002.

Of the children who lived with just one parent, in 1960 only 4.2 percent of their parents had never married; by 1980 that figure had more than tripled to 14.6 percent, and it reached 30.6 percent in 1990.

DID YOU KNOW?

Number of Children Involved in Divorce, 1950–1980

This table demonstrates the dramatic changes that took place after the middle of the 20th century.

Year	Number of divorces (thousands)	Children under 18 involved in divorce (thousands)
1950	385	299
1955	377	347
1960	393	463
1965	479	630
1970	708	870
1975	1,036	1,123
1976	1,083	1,117
1977	1,091	1,095
1978	1,130	1,147
1979	1,181	1,181
1980	1,189	1,174

Source: United States Dept. of Education, National Center for Education Statistics, from U.S. Census Bureau reports, 1996.

In other words, in 1990 several million kids were living with an "unwed" mother or father, a status which most people had considered disgraceful just one generation earlier.

REASONS FOR THE CHANGE

Historians and sociologists have come up with numerous possible causes for the dramatic increase in divorce in the 1980s and 1990s. A few of the theories are presented here.

Legal reasons

In the 1960s and 1970s, nearly every state introduced some version of no-fault divorce. In practical terms, for the first time in history, nearly any husband or wife who wanted to end his or her marriage could do so, at least from a legal point of view. These legal changes almost certainly contributed to the increase in divorce in the following years, as people who felt trapped in unhappy marriages seized the opportunity to leave them.

Economic reasons

Without the rising prosperity of the decades after World War II, many couples might not have been able to consider divorce. Greater prosperity meant people could afford to pay for divorce and could maintain two separate households thereafter. With prosperity, many Americans also came to believe that personal fulfillment and happiness were worthwhile goals in themselves. There have always been some unhappy marriages; now, perhaps, people were less willing to tolerate them.

Religious reasons

In the early 1900s, many people in troubled marriages turned to the clergy for advice. Religious leaders in most faiths tended to encourage people to stay married. Responsibility to spouse and children was thought to be more important than an individual's personal fulfillment.

Today, in contrast, people often turn to secular marriage counselors and psychotherapists for help. Many of these professionals do not believe that every marriage must be kept intact. Today's clergymen and clergywomen may feel the same way; in fact, many of them are now trained in counseling skills at secular universities.

Gender roles

The changing role of the sexes probably contributed to the rise in divorce as well. Many careers and professions that were closed to women began to open up starting in the 1970s, and the percentage of married women who worked outside the home soared. A woman who already worked outside the home, whose children were either at school or in day care, was perhaps more likely to consider divorce as a viable alternative.

In addition, by the 1970s American men were somewhat more involved in child-raising activities than their fathers had been, and courts were less likely to award **sole physical custody** of children to mothers. Since fathers no longer feared they would lose their children, they were perhaps more willing to file for divorce.

Values

Changes in popular ideas about sexual morality also had their impact on marriage. Until roughly the 1970s, few women in the United States were willing to live openly with a man outside of marriage for fear of being condemned by family and friends. Unmarried women who gave birth often gave up the child for adoption.

Following a dramatic change in popular attitudes and values in the 1960s and 1970s, the stigma against sex outside marriage became much weaker. Young people whose main goal used to be finding and keeping a husband or wife no longer felt as much pressure to get married or to stay married.

People were getting married later as well. In 1965, according to a 2003 Census Bureau report, women were on average 20.6 years old when they first married; men were 22.8. By 1985 the average age rose to 23.3 for women and 25.5 for men. In 2002, the corresponding ages were 25.3 and 26.9.

WHAT OF THE FUTURE?

Will the trend that led to higher rates of divorce continue indefinitely? The evidence is mixed, but some countertrends have appeared in recent years. At the very least, one can safely say that the trend has been leveling off, in light of the following evidence:

- Both the **crude divorce rate** (per 1,000 individuals) and the **refined divorce rate** (per 1,000 married women) have been falling steadily since around 1980.
- According to a 2001 Census Bureau report, the number of children living with both biological parents increased from 51 to 56 percent in the early 1990s. That 5 percent change adds up to about 7 million children.

- Surveys show that today's kids, even those who went through more than one divorce, expect to get married and expect to *stay* married once they do.

- More than half of all couples who live together for at least five years eventually wind up getting married, according to a July 2002 study issued by the National Center for Health Statistics of the Centers for Disease Control and Prevention.

It does seem unlikely that Americans will ever go back to the "good old days" of few divorces, as long as the no-fault laws remain on the books—and few Americans seem to want that to change. On the other hand, as Americans gradually adjust to changes in the economy, the role of the sexes, and sexual morality, marriage may become more predictable, and perhaps more stable. Only time, and the next generation, will tell.

TEENS SPEAK

Is Our Generation Different?

Wanda and Carol are friends who attend the same middle school in southern Illinois. They recently talked about the future of marriage—and divorce.

Wanda: My parents were divorced when I was just four years old. We hardly ever saw my dad after that, and my mother didn't get married again for nine years. It was really scary sometimes. Trust me, my brother Clarence and I know what divorce is like for little kids, and I'm not going to put *my* kids through that. The next generation will get the benefit of our own experience.

Carol: I hope you're right, Wanda. My best friend when I was a little girl had parents who were divorced. She used to sleep over all the time because she hated it at her own place; she said she wished my parents had had her and not her own. Her older brother George even ran away from home, it was so bad.

But guess what? Last year George got divorced himself after being married for less than a year. You can never tell what life is going to deal you.

Wanda: I'm not saying that divorce will disappear into thin air. But people like me have one goal: Don't get married till you find the right boy, and then fight like hell to make it work out. And wait till you're ready. My mom made me promise: I will hold out to 21, at least.

Carol: Well, I hope we both get lucky.

See also: Divorce, The Legal Process of

FURTHER READING

Basch, Norma. *Framing American Divorce: From the Revolutionary Generation to the Victorians)*. Berkeley, CA: University of California Press, 1999.

Goode, William J. *World Changes in Divorce Patterns*. New Haven, CT: Yale University Press, 1993.

Whitehead, Barbara Dafoe. *The Divorce Culture: Rethinking our Commitments to Marriage and Family*. New York: Vintage Books, 1996.

■ DIVORCE, THE BUSINESS SIDE OF

The financial matters that married people need to deal with when they get divorced, known as the business side of a divorce. In a sense, a marriage is a business owned by two people. When it is dissolved, the owners have to take care of a great many details, including the division of assets (all the property and goods they own) and liabilities (all the money they owe). They must also set up two new households in place of the old one.

Many of these financial matters are covered as part of the **divorce settlement**, an official document filed in court that also deals with custody and support. Married people who consider getting a divorce should pay careful attention to all these issues before making any decisions, as their future lives and living standards may be at stake.

PROPERTY AND INVESTMENTS

Unless a couple has been married for a very short period of time or have no assets, the division of property is an important part of a divorce agreement. Property can include houses, cars, furniture, valuables, a business or professional practice, collectibles, bank accounts, long-term savings, pensions and retirement plans, life insurance policies, and other assets.

A couple thinking of divorce needs to list all of these items, estimate their value, and decide how they are to be divided. For example, should movable property like a car or furniture be valued based on the current market price or based on **replacement value** (the amount it would cost to purchase a new one)? Should the couple try to put a value on an attorney's license or the **goodwill** of a business (its reputation and customer base), if the other spouse supported the family while the business or professional practice was built?

The couple needs to list their debts as well. If both names are on the home mortgage, for example, who will be primarily responsible for payments after the divorce? Who was primarily responsible for charging the money owed on the couple's credit cards, and who will pay it off?

Often the hardest part is deciding who will get what. One spouse may want to stay in the family home. He or she may have to buy out the other partner, perhaps taking out a second mortgage to carry the cost. In other cases, the couple may sell the house and divide any profits. They may agree to divide all joint property 50–50, or one party may allow the other party a higher percentage to compensate for lower expected income in the future.

Once the parties have agreed to a settlement and it is formalized in court, the couple or their representatives have to do the legal work of removing names from bank accounts, investments, and property registries; transferring funds; and physically moving assets. It is not only a tiresome, detailed process but also an emotional one. Once the last signature is placed on the last dotted line, the marriage is officially over.

INSURANCE

Generally, one or both parties to a divorce has to deal with reduced income. He or she may be in no position to handle unexpected expenses, such as medical emergencies, disabling accidents, or death in the family. Unfortunately, he or she may be caught without insurance coverage just when it is needed most.

Health insurance

Most adult Americans get their health insurance through their job or their spouse's job. During the long divorce process, anyone who is relying on a spouse's health insurance might want to contact the insurance company directly to make sure the coverage continues.

Many states have made it illegal to change a health insurance policy until a divorce is final. Once the divorce goes into effect, a spouse can usually get insurance from his or her ex-partner's company for 18 months under the federal COBRA law, which regulates employee benefits. A divorce agreement should specify what each partner is expected to pay for the children's insurance in the future and for medical, dental, or therapy bills that an insurance policy might not cover.

Life and disability insurance
Some life insurance policies gradually accumulate cash value, which can be withdrawn if the policy is canceled—for example, during a divorce. This value is usually included among the assets listed in the divorce settlement.

If the divorce settlement requires one spouse to provide spousal support or child support for a period of time, that spouse would be wise to have a life insurance policy that would cover those payments if he or she died or became disabled. The divorce settlement can include this provision too.

WILLS AND LIVING WILLS
Despite the repeated warnings of lawyers and accountants, millions of adults do not have a will. After a divorce, wills become even more important, especially for the spouse who has primary responsibility for the children. In the event of death, the executor named in the will can quickly move to protect the children's financial rights and implement that parent's wishes with regard to raising the kids.

If a couple has drawn up wills in the past, they almost always need to be changed as a result of a divorce, perhaps as soon as one partner files the **divorce petition** (the official paper that starts the process off). If someone can't bear to live with a spouse, he or she probably doesn't want that spouse to inherit hard-earned assets.

People should also look at other documents they may have signed in the past, such as **powers of attorney** and **living wills**, which give legal authority to another person if the signer becomes incapacitated. During marriage, the other person named is usually the spouse; after divorce, that probably should change.

PENSIONS AND SOCIAL SECURITY

By law and by explicit choice, most husbands and wives have a financial interest in their partner's future retirement benefits: pensions, 401Ks, IRAs, and the like. If the couple divorces before retirement, it usually makes sense to get an expert to calculate the present value of the pension, or at least that part of the pension that was accumulated during the marriage. The couple adds that amount to the list of property to be divided. Sometimes a pension plan pays out a lump sum to the divorcing spouse.

The Social Security system pays a one-half pension to a worker's spouse when the spouse reaches retirement age, unless the spouse's own pension is higher. Divorce does not cancel this right. If a person gets divorced and remarries, both the former and the current spouse are entitled to the pension. The military pension system follows similar rules.

DEBTS, CREDIT CARDS, AND BANKRUPTCY

Debts (money owed) can be a major complication in divorce. Each spouse remains solely responsible for any money that he or she borrowed (from a bank, credit card company, or private individual) *before* the marriage. However, both spouses are equally responsible for money that was borrowed while they were married; some states even hold the spouses responsible for debts incurred after the couple separates but before the divorce takes legal effect.

The divorce settlement can assign these debts to one party or the other, but anyone who is owed money can demand it from either spouse, even after the divorce, no matter what the settlement says. The only people bound by the divorce settlement are the two ex-spouses who sign it. Third parties such as banks retain all their rights. To avoid this problem, lawyers advise couples to pay off their debts *before* the divorce.

Unfortunately, many people are so impoverished by divorce that they are forced to go into **bankruptcy** (a legal process that protects people who cannot pay their debts). Bankruptcy wipes out most debts, but at a cost—a bankrupt individual may find it difficult to borrow money or get credit. He or she may be barred from certain jobs. By federal law, bankruptcy does *not* wipe out the obligations of divorce, such as spousal support and child support.

PRENUPTIAL AGREEMENTS

If a couple signed a **prenuptial agreement** ("prenup" for short) before they got married, they probably can avoid much of the conflict and confusion of divorce. A prenup is a legally binding contract that defines exactly what will happen to all property in case of divorce—including property that is acquired during the marriage. If a couple desires, they can put a time limit on the prenup; for example, they may agree that once the marriage passes the 10-year mark, the contract will no longer apply.

In order to be enforced by a court, the prenup has to cover every asset and liability of each spouse, and it cannot be unfair to either party as judged by reasonable standards. Apart from property, a prenup also can provide for marital responsibilities, style of parenting, and any other item the couple wants to include.

Few couples signed prenuptial agreements in the past, apart from the very rich. Even today brides and grooms tend to be optimistic people; few of them think of divorce before they even take their vows. However, the growth in divorce among all classes and social groups has made prenups more popular in recent years. People who have experienced a painful and expensive divorce, and who thus may be a bit less optimistic about the future, are the ones most likely to take this route.

Attorney Arlene Dubin wrote in her 2001 book *Prenups for Lovers* that the number of prenups increased fivefold between 1980 and 2000. She estimated that 20 percent of all couples getting married signed prenuptial agreements in recent years. Dubin recommends prenups in particular for people who have children from a previous marriage, own a business or hold a professional license, plan to attend professional school during the marriage, or expect an inheritance.

A couple often "strengthens the relationship" by working together on a prenup, according to Dubin. The process forces couples to be honest about their finances and their future hopes and dreams.

Couples who divorce after a long marriage or who are fortunate to have property or other assets may need to spend time and effort on the business of divorce. It may not be difficult to add up the numbers, but it can be much more challenging to divide the total in a way that both parties consider fair.

See also: Child Support, Spousal Support; Divorce, The Legal Process of; Finances and Divorce

FURTHER READING
Blum, Stephanie I., and Marc Robinson. *Divorce and Finances: Know Your Rights Clearly and Quickly.* New York: Dorling Kindersley, 2000.

Dubin, Arlene. *Prenups for Lovers.* New York: Villard, 2001.
Strauss, Steven D. *Divorce and Child Custody.* New York: W.W. Norton & Co., 1998.

■ DIVORCE, THE LEGAL PROCESS OF

The laws and procedures a couple must follow to get a divorce. For all concerned—children as well as husband and wife—divorce is a difficult experience. Fortunately for kids, though, they can usually avoid getting directly involved in one of the most unpleasant aspects: the legal process.

While divorce has become much easier in the United States over the last 30 years, "easy" is a relative term. In most states before 1970, a wife or husband seeking a divorce had to prove before the court that the other spouse had committed adultery, physical violence, or mental cruelty. Compared with that ordeal, the process is easier today. In fact, just about any spouse who wants a divorce can get one.

However, the process can still be long and expensive, especially if the marriage is more than a few years old or children are involved. Every couple who decides to divorce needs to carefully examine all the options and choose the method that is the least troublesome and gets the best results for everyone concerned.

Q & A ─────────────────────────

Question: How much does divorce cost?

Answer: According to a Utah State University report in 2003, the average couple who divorces in the United States pays about $18,000 in direct costs. Apart from legal fees, which vary greatly, that figure includes lost time at work and relocation expenses.

Federal and state government agencies also pay a high price. According to the Utah report, each divorce costs state and federal agencies approximately $30,000. That figure includes child support enforcement and temporary assistance to divorced families.

WHY DO WE NEED THE LAW?

If you and your girlfriend or boyfriend decide to break up, you do not hire a lawyer or file papers in family court. You tell your friends, "it's over," and move on. Why is divorce different?

The law gives husbands and wives many rights and responsibilities concerning property and finances, mutual support, taxation, and parental duties. When a marriage is over, all of these rights and responsibilities come into question. They must be resolved in a legally binding **divorce settlement.**

A settlement gives specific instructions on how to divide property; who (if anyone) will provide monthly support payments to the other spouse and/or the children; what the payments should be; where the children (or the parents) will live; and how much time each parent will spend with the children.

If everybody involved had the same idea of what "fair" meant, laws might not be necessary. However, that rarely happens, so the government provides legal guidelines, whether written in state laws or modified and expanded by judges through their individual decisions. If the couple cannot come to an agreement voluntarily, ultimately the courts do it for them based on these guidelines.

HOW TO REACH A SETTLEMENT

All states today allow for **no-fault divorce,** in which neither husband nor wife needs to prove that the other spouse did anything wrong. All that is needed is for one spouse to claim the marriage is "irretrievably broken" or that there are "irreconcilable differences."

About three dozen states still allow for **fault divorce.** In a fault divorce, the **plaintiff**—the spouse who is suing—must prove in court that the **defendant**—the other spouse—was unfaithful, violent, or cruel. If the judge rules for the plaintiff, the court penalizes the party at fault when drawing up the settlement.

The large majority of divorces today are no-fault. Most petitioners realize there is no way to predict how a judge will rule; if the judge fails to be convinced by the evidence, he or she can penalize the plaintiff in drawing up the settlement.

Even in a **no-fault divorce,** however, one spouse has to file a **divorce petition** in court, a document stating his or her reasons for wanting a divorce and naming the other spouse as **respondent.** In a fault case, the other spouse is the defendant.

The court delivers the petition to the respondent, who generally has 30 days to file a response, which opens the case. Practically speaking, the no-fault respondent has no right to refuse the divorce; only the petitioner can stop the process by withdrawing the petition.

Once the case is opened, the **discovery** process begins. Both parties try to "discover" exactly what properties each spouse owns, separately or together. From this point on, the couple can take one of three paths to arrive at a divorce settlement:

1. Each spouse can hire a lawyer to represent him or her in negotiations and, if need be, in a court trial before a judge; each lawyer is expected to protect the best interests of his or her client only.

2. The couple can try to cooperate in reaching an agreement, with the help of divorce professionals such as mediators.

3. The couple can make their own agreement, using consultants when appropriate, and file papers directly with the courts; this is usually called a **do-it-yourself divorce**.

Let the lawyers negotiate—or litigate

The lawyer method is usually called adversarial, because each client/lawyer team is the adversary or opponent of the other side. As a rule, the adversarial method is the most expensive.

In many cases using a lawyer may be unavoidable. When a good deal of property is involved, such as a family business, it may be worth paying for legal advice so that each side can be confident of getting a fair deal.

Couples typically resort to adversarial lawyers if neither party trusts the other, or if both parties are too angry to cooperate. Also, if one spouse is less knowledgeable about legal and financial matters, or has a less forceful personality, that spouse should probably consider hiring a lawyer to ensure they get a fair deal.

Everyone is familiar with "lawyer jokes," whose premise is that the legal profession is interested only in making money by exploiting human suffering. No doubt some attorneys (another word for lawyers) fall into that category, but in family law at least, experienced attorneys usually advise their clients to be cooperative and reasonable. They know that when a settlement ignores the needs of one of the parties, it can hurt the children and might even backfire against the best interests of the "winning" party. Of course, when a husband or wife is anxious to "get even" or "punish" the other party, they may deliberately hire a ruthless attorney.

Even when lawyers are involved, the divorcing couple does not necessarily wind up in **litigation**, or adversarial proceedings in court. In fact, formal divorce trials are not common. A study of over 1,000 divorces in California involving children, reported in the journal *The Future of Children* in 1994, found that 80 percent of the couples reached a voluntary settlement on their own or with the help of their attorneys. Court-ordered mediation and formal custody evaluations took care of most of the remaining cases. Only 3.5 percent of the 1,000 divorces were ever argued before a judge.

Mediation and collaborative divorce

The average adversarial divorce can cost between $10,000 and $30,000. **Mediation** is much less expensive. When it works, it can also save a great deal of fighting and turmoil.

With mediation, the couple is the joint client of one or two neutral professional mediators, who can be social workers or attorneys. The mediator or team suggests options, encourages brainstorming, and pushes the two parties toward compromise. Sometimes a financial or tax consultant is brought into the process to clarify information. All of the professionals agree in advance that they will not testify if the case winds up in court, thus allowing the couple to speak freely.

Many courts provide mediation services, sometimes at a modest fee. Some judges may order a litigating couple to use such services, which offer advice and conclusions that the judges often accept. Mediation probably works best if both partners want the divorce, if both intend to play a major parenting role, and, of course, if they trust or respect one another.

Is mediation better than litigation? Experts disagree. Famed psychologist Judith Wallerstein reported in her 2000 book *The Unexpected Legacy of Divorce* that "most parents [in her 25-year longitudinal study of over 100 families] find the mediation helpful and reassuring," and are more likely to abide by mediated settlements. On the other hand, psychologist E. Mavis Hetherington reported in her 2002 book, *For Better or For Worse,* that women in her own longitudinal study of several hundred families were less satisfied than men with mediated settlements, which, in her view, tend to give fathers a greater parenting role than courts do.

Based on the people in her study, Wallerstein believes that the choice of mediation or litigation does not affect the way children adjust to a divorce. She attributes this to the fact that neither path brings children directly into the process. Since their opinions are not usually sought, she believes, their needs are not always met.

Another, fairly recent option is **collaborative divorce**, which is now available in many states. In this approach, each spouse has an attorney, as in the adversarial route, but all parties agree in advance to work in a cooperative spirit and avoid litigation.

Any expert or specialist who is consulted in a collaborative divorce is considered to be working for both parties. If the case does wind up in court, the attorneys and consultants will not testify. The parties usually pledge to aim for a quick resolution of custody issues.

This option can be useful for people with complicated or disputed issues that require the expertise of dedicated attorneys but who are still able to keep their emotions under control.

Do-it-yourself

Some people like to be self-sufficient. They do their own plumbing, sewing, painting, and cooking. With some divorces, it is possible to be your own lawyer too.

Publishers have developed a library of books, manuals, and kits for do-it-yourself divorces, with different versions for each state (and in some states, for each county). Some lawyers advise couples to take this route, provided both spouses agree to the divorce, the marriage is only a few years old, and no children or substantial assets are involved.

Fact Or Fiction?

You can save a lot of money during divorce if you do the legal work yourself.

Fact: If a couple has been married for only a few years, if they do not own a house or other property, and if neither is in debt, then they probably will save money by acting as "their own lawyer." But when a couple has been married for several years or more, owns a home, business, or property, or owes money, it may be a case of "penny wise, pound foolish" to try to save on legal fees. At the very least, each partner should consult a knowledgeable lawyer to make sure he or she is not unfairly treated in the divorce settlement.

Some local courts provide consultants to help explain the procedures and the forms. In many areas, small private agencies provide that service for a fee. In either case, the entire process may cost just a few hundred dollars. However, this route may not be a good idea if either partner suspects the other of hiding assets or is unclear as to his or her rights.

DEALING WITH LAWYERS

Finding the right lawyer for a divorce can take time, but it is worth the effort. Every lawyer has a unique combination of experience, style, and personality that may or may not meet the needs of a particular client or case.

An attorney who has worked successfully for a friend or relative is often the best bet. On the other hand, friends may have had different goals in their divorces. One may want a tough fighter, while another wants someone who favors compromise.

Local bar associations (lawyers' organizations) can help individuals find a family lawyer. Private referral services, which get a fee for each referral, may not be as reliable.

Before hiring an attorney, one should interview him or her in person—no payment should be required for that initial discussion. It is an opportunity to assess the attorney and learn about his or her fees. The attorney can also provide an estimate of how long the process will take and possible outcomes based on similar cases in the area. He or she should also be willing to answer any questions or clear up any confusion the prospective client might have.

Divorce lawyers may charge from $100 an hour to much more. In complicated cases, or when the client prolongs the case by holding out for a better settlement than the lawyer thinks likely, fees could reach tens of thousands of dollars. Simpler cases, where the two ex-spouses are reasonable, might cost as little as a few thousand dollars.

VARYING STATE LAWS

In the United States divorce is controlled primarily by the states. Before the no-fault era began around 1970, substantial differences existed among the states in regard to grounds for divorce and in property settlements.

Those differences have largely disappeared. As a result, few people cross state lines or national borders to get a divorce. Even if they do, their divorce is usually not considered valid in their home state unless the other spouse consents.

Divorce laws in nine states follow the principle of **community property**. The other 41 states are called common law states. In community property states, joint property is divided 50–50 in the divorce settlement. Joint property includes nearly all income that either spouse received while the marriage was in effect and nearly all property purchased by either party during the marriage.

Legal Grounds for Divorce, by State

The first two columns show whether the state has a no-fault approach or it still allows for "traditional" fault divorce as well. The next two columns show the major reasons a plaintiff can present to justify the divorce before the court.

State	No fault	No fault & traditional	Incompatible	Living separately	State	No fault	No fault & traditional	Incompatible	Living separately
Alabama		X	X	X	Montana	X		X	X
Alaska	X		X	X	Nebraska	X			
Arizona	X	X			Nevada			X	X
Arkansas		X		X	New Hampshire		X		X
California	X				New Jersey		X		X
Colorado		X			New Mexico		X	X	
Connecticut		X		X	New York		X		X
Delaware		X	X	X	North Carolina		X		X
Dist. Columbia	X			X	North Dakota		X		
Florida	X				Ohio		X	X	X
Georgia		X			Oklahoma			X	
Hawaii				X	Oregon	X			
Idaho		X			Pennsylvania		X		X
Illinois		X		X	Rhode Island		X		X
Indiana			X		South Carolina		X		X
Iowa	X				South Dakota		X		
Kansas			X		Tennessee		X		X
Kentucky	X			X	Texas		X		X
Louisiana		X		X	Utah		X		X
Maine		X			Vermont		X		X
Maryland		X		X	Virginia		X		X
Massachusetts		X			Washington	X			
Michigan	X				West Virginia		X		X
Minnesota	X				Wisconsin	X			
Mississippi		X			Wyoming			X	X
Missouri		X		X					

Source: American Bar Association, 2004.

In the common-law states, sometimes called **equitable distribution** states, the courts generally grant property to the person whose name is on the asset. However, judges have considerable leeway and can take into account the length of marriage as well as the age, health, and economic situation of each partner in trying to reach a fair division of property.

WHO'S ON WHOSE SIDE?

In an adversarial divorce and even in a collaborative one, each spouse can be sure that at least one person is looking out for his or her interests. By contrast, in the various types of mediation the professionals try *not* to take sides. Most people can count on allies outside the process for support—their relatives, friends, or colleagues.

The one place each spouse should *not* seek allies is among the children. Unfortunately, as experts who study and write about divorce warn, each parent may often be tempted to try to win the children over to his or her side.

TEENS SPEAK

I Am Not Your Lawyer!

Michael's parents have been in the process of getting a divorce for over a year. It has become so stressful for the 15-year-old only boy that he has actually mailed his parents the following letter complaining of their behavior. He wrote:

"Dear Mother and Father. Somehow you both got me mixed up with someone else, so I am writing to remind you that I am not your lawyer. I do not know anything about pensions and IRAs, and I am not interesting in knowing about them. I do not know anything about mortgages and credit histories either.

"I know you both want the best for me, but please try to figure it all out by yourselves; it is too much to ask a high school sophomore to be judge and jury for his own parents. As far as I am concerned, you are both wrong, so that's what I will tell you from now on if you ask.

> "If you both keep complaining to me about what you deserve and what the other one owes you, I will start sending you a bill for my services, since you are keeping me from doing my homework.
>
> "Yours truly, your son and not your lawyer, Michael."

Such behavior is unfair to kids. Children of divorce face enough problems without being dragged into adult disputes, which they may not even understand. Children will eventually make their own judgments about each parent *as a parent*, which is all that should matter anyway.

See also: Divorce in America; Finances and Divorce

FURTHER READING
McKay, Matthew, Peter Rogers, Joan Blades, et al. *The Divorce Book.* Oakland, CA: New Harbinger Publications, Inc., 1999.
Strauss, Steven D. *Divorce and Child Custody.* New York: W.W. Norton & Co., 1998.

■ DIVORCE, THE PSYCHOLOGICAL COST FOR SPOUSES

The emotional impact that a divorce has on both partners. People usually seek a divorce because they are depressed, unfulfilled, resentful, or anxious in their marriage. They may assume the divorce can eliminate those feelings, but relief does not automatically come.

Divorce itself can be a source of new problems and pressures, even for the spouse who first wanted it. The other spouse, who may have found the marriage acceptable or even satisfying, may feel even more stressed and unhappy during and after the divorce.

Q & A

Question: Are people happier after divorce?

Answer: Experts disagree. It is very hard to measure happiness scientifically. Besides, how can you average out a happy person and an unhappy person?

Surveys, interviews, and observations suggest that a *majority* of divorced people are happier than they were when married. The surveys were conducted in the period immediately after divorce and again at intervals of several years. The Virginia Longitudinal Study of Divorce and Remarriage, conducted by E. Mavis Hetherington between 1972 and 1992, found that more adults benefited from divorce in the long term.

On the other hand, a study published in 2002 by sociologist Linda Waite reached the opposite conclusion based on data from the university-based National Survey of Family and Households. The study interviewed 645 people who said they were unhappily married, and conducted follow-up interviews with the same people five years later. Those who were divorced were no happier than those who had remained married, using twelve different signs of psychological well-being. Even those who had remarried after divorce were no happier. Furthermore, of those who remained married, nearly 80 percent of the unhappiest adults had turned around within five years and now considered their marriages to be happy.

In the months immediately following divorce, most people experience emotional pain. They also face practical challenges resulting from disrupted lives, new financial pressures, a greater workload outside the home, and uncertainty about future living arrangements for themselves and their children.

Either spouse may also feel some combination of anger, loneliness, anxiety, depression, or guilt. Often, newly divorced people feel unattractive or unsuccessful, and they may exhibit inconsistent or unstable behavior. They may have mood swings, paying inconsistent attention to their surroundings and even their children.

Most people eventually overcome these problems. Even so, people who think they may want a divorce should take into account the psychological cost that the process almost always brings.

DISRUPTION, OVERWORK, AND ANXIETY

Any change to a person's routine can cause stress. Divorce can overturn the entire routine almost overnight, even affecting an individual's self-image or sense of identity.

Being a partner in a marriage is a crucial part of a person's identity. Without that identity, some people lose self-confidence in day-to-day social interactions. In addition, they may no longer fit into their circle of married friends. Some friends withdraw for fear of getting involved in the conflict. Thus a divorced man or woman may lose the support of friends just when they are needed most.

Some identity issues can be particularly damaging to divorced women. Husbands are more likely to work outside the home than wives. When both work, the man's job is likely to have a higher social status than the woman's, even today. If so, some of that higher status may have been shared with the wife. After the divorce, the man loses his status as a husband but retains the prestige that goes along with his job. The woman may lose the shared prestige of both identities.

Divorced men, on the other hand, face a different problem. They tend to be less familiar with domestic tasks and are often overwhelmed by the need to set up and maintain a household. Sometimes they have difficulty feeling that their ill-maintained bachelor quarters are really a home.

Because fathers are less likely to have **primary physical custody** (children usually spend the bulk of their time with their mothers after divorce), divorced men are at greater risk of feeling lonely and depressed. On the other hand, according to E. Mavis Hetherington in her 2002 book, *For Better or For Worse*, and other researchers as well, divorced men are more likely to stay connected with married friends than their ex-wives are.

Hetherington attributes that connection among men to two factors: when their children visit, men tend to invite other kids (accompanied by their parents) to entertain them. And, divorced women are sometimes excluded from married circles because married women may see them as potential rivals. In addition, divorced men are more likely to get help with housework and other chores from girlfriends than their ex-wives receive from boyfriends.

Whatever stresses may exist in a marriage, people tend to find comfort in household routines and think of their home as a refuge from outside pressures. These very routines tend to fall apart following divorce. At least one spouse is living in a new home; even the spouse living in the old home may be spending less time there and more time working outside to make up for lost income. Many child-related routines come undone as well, as kids move back and forth between parents and parental discipline weakens amid all the disruption.

Deprived of comforting routines, many recently divorced people feel adrift, unfocused, and anxious. **Anxiety** (a feeling of unease and fear) can in turn make people irritable. It can also lower people's resistance and send them to the doctor with real or sometimes exaggerated ailments. Hetherington reports a large increase in doctors' visits in the first year following divorce.

Many divorced men and women are burdened with an increased workload both at home and outside the home. Two households are more expensive to maintain than one, and someone has to pay the price. Often both parties to the divorce must work extra hours or get second jobs to cover the difference. Keeping house also requires labor—shopping, cooking, cleaning, painting, gardening, and making repairs. Where once these tasks may have been shared, now they are duplicated. The additional workload can lead to physical and mental exhaustion.

POOR SELF-CONFIDENCE, LONELINESS, AND ANGER

Very few people are able to ignore the judgments of others. When their life partner—the person who presumably knows them best—rejects them, their self-esteem is bound to suffer.

TEENS SPEAK

Even the Tough Can Cry

Thirteen-year-old twins Tiffany and Karyn never thought they would see their mother cry. Tiffany explained, "Mom was always so tough. Nothing fazed her. Once we had a car accident and she was laid up for weeks; but even in the hospital she was always laughing and cracking jokes."

Karyn agreed. "That's what made it so scary this time. At first when Dad moved out and they told us they were splitting up, she was the same old Mom—you know, 'When the going gets tough, the tough go shopping.' But suddenly I went in the kitchen and she was crying."

"At first I didn't believe Karyn," Tiffany said, "until I saw it myself. Every night almost, she would just break out crying. The first time I ran over and hugged her, but she pushed me away, like she was contagious or something and didn't want us to catch it."

Luckily for their mom, the girls were so scared they decided to take action on their own. They talked to their

> grandparents, who looked up programs for divorced moms, and insisted that their daughter talk to a counselor about her feelings.
>
> "She still gets real sad, sometimes," Tiffany says, "but now she lets us help her get over the bad patches. Last night we all made lasagna together."
>
> "And after that, she made us clean up our room," said Karyn. "She hadn't even stuck her head in for weeks. That's when I knew the old mom was back."

Insecurities about personal appearance often come to the surface. Married people, especially those with children, usually do not have time to keep up with the latest clothing fads or maintain a perfect body. After divorce, they may feel less than desirable to the opposite sex. Loneliness may encourage them to seek romantic involvements, but they are now older and more burdened by responsibilities than when they were single years before. Many lack social confidence.

Divorced parents also may feel guilty when they begin to date, afraid that their social life will detract from parenting. But many therapists say that on the contrary, parents are better able to help their children if they can manage to take one evening a week off to pamper themselves.

People who divorce are often consumed with a sense of failure. They could not get their marriage—usually the most important fact of their life—to succeed. With time they may recognize that the marriage was not a total failure, but the negative memories usually dominate at the start. In some cases this sense of failure and low self-image can even carry over to people's jobs.

Divorced people, especially in the first year or two, often feel a void (empty space) in their emotional lives, the space once filled by their ex-spouse. That may be true even with spouses who argued and fought. The custodial parent who lives with the children most of the time may get company and comfort from them but may also feel lonely for adult companionship.

Loneliness, a sense of failure, and self-pity can reinforce one another in an unhealthy cycle. These feelings often turn into anger at the spouse who "put me into this situation."

Anger can have a positive impact. It is one way of escaping depression. It can also energize people for the hard tasks they must face and motivate people to succeed in their new lives as the "best revenge."

On the other hand, severe anger can be unhealthy. It can distort people's sense of judgment. Therapists advise people not to make important decisions while angry. If anger, anxiety, or depression do not subside with time after a divorce, people should consider visiting a professional therapist or joining a support group. The goal should be to move on to a more productive, satisfying phase of life.

Fact Or Fiction?

The "left" spouse (the one whose partner wanted the marriage to end) will always be the unhappy one.

Fact: The left spouse may indeed be very unhappy at the start of the process. But, according to E. Mavis Hetherington, citing her study in *For Better or For Worse,* "by the end of the second year, there were few differences between those left and 'leavers.'"

Those who are left behind may be spared the feelings of guilt, failure, and regret that leavers often report. Besides, they usually benefit from the sympathy of friends, family, and workmates.

The real danger for "left" spouses is that they may continue to dwell on feelings of resentment and anger, sometimes for years. Psychologists say they may wind up feeling helpless to change their situation. However badly they may have been treated, the therapists say, eventually it is necessary to put the past where it belongs—in the past.

See also: Children, Psychological Effects of Divorce on; Communications and Compromise in Divorced Families

FURTHER READING
McKay, Matthew, Peter Rogers, Joan Blades, et al. *The Divorce Book.* Oakland, CA: New Harbinger Publications, Inc., 1999.

■ FAMILIES, BLENDED
Stepfamilies; families formed as a result of marriages that involve children from previous relationships.

Blended families play a significant role in American life today. In fact, the U.S. Census Bureau reported in 2001 that 17 percent of the nation's children in 1996 were living in blended families; the figures are believed to be about the same today.

In 1996 more than 5 million children were living with one biological parent and one stepparent, and 2.1 million were living with **stepsiblings** (a son or daughter of a stepparent). About 7.8 million children lived with **half siblings** (brothers or sisters who shared one biological

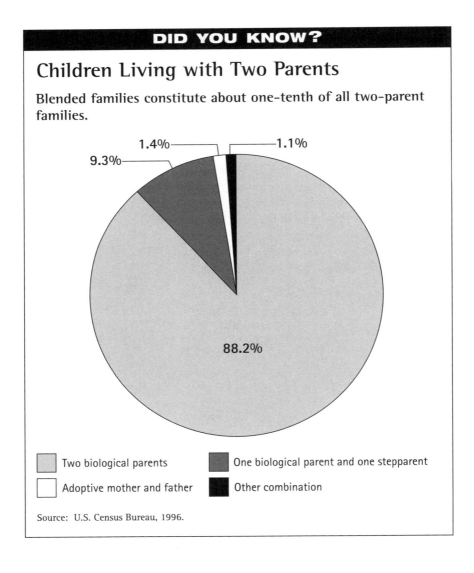

DID YOU KNOW?

Children Living with Two Parents

Blended families constitute about one-tenth of all two-parent families.

1.4%   1.1%
9.3%

88.2%

☐ Two biological parents   ■ One biological parent and one stepparent
☐ Adoptive mother and father   ■ Other combination

Source: U.S. Census Bureau, 1996.

parent). Blended families constitute about one-tenth of all two-parent families, as shown in the chart from a recent Census Bureau report.

Most blended families are created when a divorced parent remarries or moves in with another adult, but sometimes the story begins with the death of a parent. In either case, the events that broke up the original families usually leave behind a host of problems and challenges. Stepparents and stepsiblings can sometimes help a child deal with these problems, but they also can create a whole new set of problems and issues.

MERGING FAMILIES

A recent long-term study of 1,400 divorced families, reported in psychologist E. Mavis Hetherington's book *For Better or For Worse*, found that within six years of divorce, 75 percent of men and 50 percent of women remarry. For divorced people, a remarriage usually means a chance to start anew. For their children, it may mean giving up the dream that their parents will get back together. At the same time, they must deal with a stepparent and, often, stepchildren, whom they did not choose and whom they do not love. Even worse, the other parent may be hurt or angry at the remarriage, which can put a strain on any child.

The experts agree that a stepfamily almost never works the same way a **nuclear family**, which is composed of a couple and their biological children, does. Relationships between stepparents and stepchildren and among stepsiblings are rarely as close—unless the kids are very young and the biological parent is absent or has passed away. People who expect a blended family to work perfectly are likely to be disappointed.

On the other hand, adding a second parent can ease the practical and financial strains of single-parent households. And some stepparents may offer emotional and material benefits that the divorced parent was unable to provide. A stepparent can never replace a parent, but he or she can often develop into a close friend.

STEPSIBLINGS

Even in an intact nuclear family, brothers and sisters do not always get along. However, they have a few big advantages—they have known each other from birth. They know they will always be siblings, whatever changes life may bring.

In contrast, stepsiblings don't usually show up for the first time as infants; they appear as kids with personalities and habits of their own. They are likely to have their own ideas about how a family should operate. Often, new stepsiblings are reluctant to commit themselves emotionally. After all, many of them have been through their parents' divorce; they are not so sure if these new brothers and sisters are going to be in their lives for long.

Stepsiblings can have many good reasons to dislike each other. They usually have different interests, friends, and relatives. When one family moves in with the other, one group of kids has to suddenly share a home and sometimes even a room with the newcomers, while the kids moving in may resent losing their old familiar home. Sometimes stepparents "lean over backwards" to win over their new stepkids, and their own kids may be jealous of the preferential treatment. When these problems are present, kids in blended families sometimes separate into two gangs, "us against them."

Hetherington found that more than half of the children who share the same biological parents get along well at least part of the time, whether they live in intact, divorced, or blended families. By contrast, only 25 percent of stepsiblings had such positive ties. Half siblings, who shared only one biological parent, were the most likely to have hostile relationships.

If you find yourself in such a situation, the best thing to do is to be honest. Talk to your parent and your stepparent. It may take time to become friends with your stepsiblings, but talking may help you clear up misunderstandings and resolve petty conflicts that can make family life an unpleasant ordeal for everyone.

STEPPARENTS

Being a stepparent is a tough job. Stepparents have no legal responsibilities for their stepkids and no rights over them—not even the right to order emergency medical treatment. Yet everyone expects stepparents to be supportive and loving. They want their stepkids to love them, but they know they are likely to be resented for stepping into their "real" parent's shoes. It is an ambiguous role with few models to follow.

TEENS SPEAK

It Takes Time

Ari's mother was killed in an automobile crash when he was only six. His father could not take care of four children all by

himself, so the children were parceled out to various relatives in the neighborhood. After three years, Ari's father remarried. His new wife had two children of her own, and he brought his own children to live with their new stepmother.

"My stepmother is okay," Ari admitted a few months later, "but I liked it better with my Aunt Raisie, that's my mother's sister. I had my own room, but now I have to share. My new brothers don't like me either. Or anyway, they stick together all the time. The only time I have peace and quiet is when they go visit their own father. I have three sisters too."

Ari loves his aunt very much. "She used to tell us stories about my mother. My stepmother doesn't want me to talk about her. My father told me she gets hurt when I tell her what a good cook my mother was. But I can't help it, it's the truth."

Ari's Aunt Raisie told him he should help his father by getting along with his new family, so he tries. However, the only time he really feels comfortable is when he and his sisters go to his aunt's house for lunch on Saturday afternoons.

Last week, though, his stepmother made carrot soup from a recipe his aunt taught her. "It tasted almost like my mother made," Ari said. "My sisters were all crying afterwards, but it did make me feel a little better about my stepmother."

Kids are often jealous of their new stepparents—angry that they have to share their parent with a new person and jealous on behalf of their other biological parent. Adolescents, who are usually testing the limits of parental control, may particularly resent discipline or interference from a stepparent. Even when kids come to love their stepparents, which eventually happens in many cases, they rarely worry about the stepparent the way they do their biological parents.

Problems between parents and stepchildren are one of the main reasons that second marriages fail. When kids are present, second marriages have a 50 percent higher chance of failing, according to Hetherington. Only one-third of stepfathers and one-quarter of stepmothers ever become a strong authority figure whose decisions are respected and followed by their stepkids.

Boys are more likely to welcome a new stepfather, especially if their own father is not around much. Now they won't be the only man in the household. On the other hand, girls often feel that a stepfather will get in the way of their close ties to their mother.

Some stepfathers may avoid getting close to their stepdaughters to protect against sexual feelings or accusations of misconduct. According to professor Charlotte Shoup Olsen in her 1997 book, *Stepping Stones: Building Step Relationships*, "What would be viewed by a biological family as normal affection and emotional support can easily be misinterpreted as sexual advances and inappropriate contact in stepfamilies."

Hetherington reported in *For Better or For Worse* that in her study, girls in blended families had their first periods nine months earlier on average than girls in intact families. By age 15, 65 percent of girls in divorced families had engaged in sex at least once, compared with 54 percent of girls in blended families and only 40 percent of girls in intact families.

A stepmother sometimes has an even harder job than a stepfather. Most men expect their wives to take on the work of nurturing a family and keeping order. Yet if the stepmother tries to mother her stepchildren, they and their biological mother may resent her. When a stepmother sees her stepchildren only on weekends and special occasions, she often succeeds in making friends with them. But when she is the primary custodian, Hetherington found, conflict with the nonresident biological mother can continue for years.

MULTIPLE MARRIAGES, MULTIPLE KIDS
In Hetherington's study, when parents got divorced, about 20 percent of their children developed emotional or behavior problems. When they got divorced a *second* time, the figure rose to 38 percent.

Life with a multitude of parents, ex-parents, grandparents, and other relatives can be confusing and unstable. Children in that situation often seek out a trusted adult outside the immediate family to talk to. Sometimes a relative, neighbor, teacher, or even the parent of a friend can provide the stability and impartial advice that may be lacking at home.

WHAT TO DO AND WHAT NOT TO DO
What stepfamilies need most is time—time for family members to get to know one another and learn to get along. With good communication and honesty, the new family may establish rewarding routines and traditions of its own. Families should enlist their relatives to participate as well.

Dwelling on the past will not help. A conversation that begins, "*We* always used to do it *this* way" may quickly turn into an argument. When this happens, according to psychologist Judith Wallerstein in *The Unexpected Legacy of Divorce*, "The family becomes like a battle-field or political campaign. People take sides, alliances are formed, and there is much blaming, finger-pointing, and scapegoating."

Home should be a place where people can relax and be themselves, a refuge from the pressures of work and school. With goodwill, time, and a little effort, many parents and stepparents manage to build supportive new homes for their children.

See also: Communication and Compromise in Divorced Families; Marriage Lifestyles, Alternative

FURTHER READING
Chedekel, David. *The Blended Family Sourcebook: A Guide to Negotiating Change.* Chicago, IL: Contemporary Books, 2002.
Hurwitz, Jane. *Coping in a Blended Family.* New York: Rosen Publishing Group, 1997.
O'Connor, Anne. *The Truth About Stepfamilies: Real American Stepfamilies Speak Out.* New York: Marlowe, 2003.

■ FINANCES AND DIVORCE
The impact that divorce has on the income and expenses of family members.

When people consider getting divorced, they often fail to foresee the emotional costs for themselves and their children. They should find it much simpler, however, to foresee the *financial* costs. Husband and wife can calculate whether they will be better or worse off financially after the divorce. They can also estimate the economic impact on their children.

Most people suffer financially as a result of divorce, at least in the first year or two. As time passes, people can make further decisions that impact their finances, such as remarriage or a career change. As a general rule, however, families are somewhat poorer and under greater money pressure after a divorce than they were before.

The impact of divorce on living standards varies with each family, and also may differ between husband and wife. In most cases, a

DID YOU KNOW?

Divorce and Poverty

	Men		Women	
Income	Married	Divorced	Married	Divorced
Below poverty level	10.1	9.1	11.9	20.7
Up to twice poverty level	17.3	15.5	18.0	26.7
More than twice poverty level	72.1	72.7	69.8	52.1
Not reported	0.6	2.7	0.3	0.5

Source: U.S. Census Bureau, Survey of Income and Program Participation, 1996.

woman's monthly income declines after the divorce, even if her ex-husband pays child support and spousal support. To make matters worse, the woman is usually the **primary custodial parent** (the children live with her most of the time), and cannot work the extra hours she might need to get back to her predivorce income.

The gap between the living standards of men and women may be narrowing somewhat. A 1997 study by sociologist Nicholas Wolfinger, based on data from several hundred families compiled by the National Survey of Families and Households, found that the per capita drop in income for women following a divorce was about 50 percent less than it had been ten years before. Wolfinger attributed the improvement to the greater earning power of women today. Nevertheless, he reported, divorced women were still five times more likely than divorced men to live below the federal government's poverty line.

Divorced parents often report that their children seem more upset about the material possessions they can no longer buy than about the family's emotional suffering. The children's reaction doesn't mean they don't care; they may find it easier to focus on the immediate physical losses than on the emotional pain, which usually takes longer to express and work through. Material goods can also affect teenagers' status among their friends, which doesn't make divorce any easier to bear.

ONE-TIME COSTS: LEGAL, HOME SALE, NEW HOMES

Many families encounter substantial one-time costs as a result of a divorce. These costs can cut deeply into savings. Some of these costs impact both parties, but even those expenses that only directly impact one spouse can reduce the total amount of money available for the settlement and for spousal and child support after the divorce. These expenses include:

- The cost of the divorce itself, which can range from several hundred to tens of thousands of dollars.

- The costs entailed in selling a residence and/or buying one or two new residences; typical costs run to about 8 percent of the proceeds of each sale.

- The cost of setting up at least one new household, including security deposits on rentals and at least some painting and renovation.

- The cost of setting up new financial and utility accounts.

- Furniture, housewares, and appliances to outfit at least one new residence.

- In some cases, the cost of a down payment on an additional car.

LIVING COSTS: "TWO CAN LIVE AS CHEAPLY AS ONE"

The old saying goes, "Two can live as cheaply as one." Divorce forces a rephrasing: Two households cost a lot more to keep up than one.

In almost every case, housing costs for divorced families rise substantially. Custodial parents often remain in the family home with the children. They must keep up mortgage or rental payments, even though they have lost part or all of the income provided by the noncustodial parent. The noncustodial parent must pay monthly housing costs on a separate residence, while continuing to provide some support for his or her children and former spouse.

Child care bills typically rise after a divorce, to pay for a replacement of whatever role the noncustodial parent used to play in child care. For similar reasons, divorced people may need to hire domestic and maintenance help to take care of chores that previously were shared by both spouses.

Food expenses tend to rise as well. Smaller households are less efficient in using up leftovers and perishable staples, and the chaotic schedule in many recently divorced households means that some home meals may be replaced by more costly restaurant meals or prepared food.

The total health insurance budget may be greater, too. If the couple decides to keep an existing policy for one parent, the other must buy a new policy. The cost of that policy usually is greater than the savings realized by removing one adult from the old policy, especially if an employer was paying part of the cost. The children can be insured through either parent.

Additional money may be spent on life insurance as well. An intact family often pays the cost of life insurance only for the high earner. After divorce, the custodial parent may feel the need to be insured as well.

Intact families usually save money by purchasing family memberships in fitness clubs, country clubs, churches, and a host of social, charitable, and cultural institutions. If the family wants to maintain those memberships for all family members, someone will have to pay for additional individual memberships.

Large family units are often more efficient in using cars. A family that managed with one car probably needs two after the divorce. If a family had two cars to share between parents and one or two older kids, three may well be needed after the divorce. The ongoing expenses for auto loans, insurance, repairs, and parking can be costly. If families decide to do without an extra car, they may have to budget funds for occasional taxis or public transportation.

Children as well as parents may need psychotherapy or counseling to get them through critical periods in a divorce. Even if covered by insurance, the out-of-pocket payments can be significant.

TEENS SPEAK

The Price Was High, but It Was Worth It

Most kids don't have swimming pools and professional gyms at home. That's why Jared's friends used to think he was the luckiest kid.

"Lucky? Hello?" he says now, looking back. "My older brother and I were never happy for one day living there. As far back as I can remember our parents fought like cats and dogs. Big as the house was, you could hear them screaming everywhere."

When the marriage broke up two years ago, Jared and his brothers moved with their mom to a small house two miles away. "All of a sudden it was a different world. I used to have all the money I needed. Now there's always a couple of days before my dad's check comes when we're all real stretched.

"It's cool. My brother picked up some hours pumping gas, and next year when I turn 16 he's going to get me in there too.

"We still see dad, but he finally sold the house. He says the money is all going for our college. Truth? I wouldn't want that house back anyway. What good is a pool when you're afraid to go back into the house?"

CHILD AND SPOUSAL SUPPORT

Among the biggest items in people's budgets after a divorce are child support (payments to cover children's living expenses) and spousal support (payments to cover an ex-spouse's living expenses). Unfortunately, the exact amount of support cannot be known until the final **divorce settlement** (the legal agreement that covers all financial and custody arrangements). However, experienced attorneys know the typical amounts awarded in their jurisdictions (the local area covered by a particular court) and should be able to provide good estimates.

In the past, some spouses managed to avoid or delay support payments; new laws and tougher enforcement have reduced nonpayment. Nevertheless, unlike a paycheck, support payments are likely to be late, partial, or skipped on occasion, even in the best of circumstances.

Support payments can affect a person's credit rating. Banks look at all of a person's regular obligations, including support payments, in deciding whether to grant loans and at what rates. In other words, even if a parent pays the same amount in child support that he or she used to pay for routine expenses before the divorce, the credit rating of the parent paying child support may go down. Furthermore, knowing that support checks are less reliable than paychecks, lenders may be reluctant to lend money to the parent receiving support payments as well, despite laws and banking regulations.

TAX ISSUES

The tax issues concerning marriage and divorce are complicated and can change from year to year. Congress, the Internal Revenue Service (IRS), and the courts have often tinkered with the laws in ways that cannot be predicted in advance.

The questions that must be considered before the divorce settlement is finalized include:

- Which parent should list the children as dependents?
- Which parent should take the Earned Income Credit (a payment from the government to employed low income parents)?
- Should support payments be structured as spousal support or child support?
- Will a partner's move place him or her in another city or state with different tax laws?
- How will real-estate taxes affect each spouse after divorce?
- Which parent will eventually pay capital gains tax on the property divided by the divorce?
- What would be the effect on taxes if the family's house was sold and one or both spouses moved to rental homes?

For years, tax experts have argued over the size and importance of a hidden, unintended "marriage penalty" built into the tax system. Most observers agree that as a result of the complex IRS code, there are some situations in which married people filing as a couple wind up paying more taxes than two unmarried people with similar incomes would pay.

If there is a "marriage penalty," getting a divorce should lead to a tax benefit for some couples. However, the Congressional Budget Office has reported that based on 1996 taxes, some 25 million couples got a "marriage benefit" (lower taxes as a result of being married) averaging $1,300 as opposed to only 20 million couples who were "penalized" for being married, at an average cost of $1,380. In any case, the tax gain or loss from divorce is not likely to be major, as compared with all the other costs.

COSTS OF JOINT CUSTODY

Joint physical custody (the sharing of the children's upbringing by both parents in both their homes) can create additional expenses in the postdivorce budget. Travel costs (including airfare in many cases) are the largest component of this expense. A certain amount of duplication in kids' clothing and personal effects is almost inevitable as well. Those fathers who did not spend much time with their kids before the divorce may wind up spending substantial amounts on movies, excursions, and other activities to keep their kids entertained during their periodic visits.

Although people sometimes lose track of financial issues during the emotional turmoil of divorce, the decisions they make, or fail to make, are likely to affect them and their children for years to come. The time to consider these matters is *before* the divorce takes effect.

See also: Child Support, Spousal Support; Divorce, The Business Side of; Divorce, The Legal Process of

FURTHER READING

Blum, Stephanie and Mark Robinson. *Divorce and finances.* NY: Dorling Kindersley, 2000.

McKay, Matthew, Peter Rogers, Joan Blades, et al. *The Divorce Book: A Practical and Compassionate Guide.* Oakland, CA: New Harbinger Publications, 2001.

■ GENERATIONAL PATTERNS AND ADULT CHILDREN OF DIVORCE

The long-term effect of a couple's divorce on their children's lives. Most people who live through their parents' divorce manage to work past the practical problems and eventually adapt to their new situation. Some even find that their lives are better than ever—once they get past the initial hurt and insecurity.

Do the children fully recover from the emotional effects? After all, the divorce broke up their home, pulled away their security blanket, and turned their lives upside down. Some people claim that parental divorce always leaves children with emotional scars and affects their behavior as they grow up and become adults. A Web search on **adult children of divorce** pulls up thousands of sites; many of them offer specialized counseling and therapy for people who feel that a childhood divorce continues to harm them as adults.

The research done so far, however, does not confirm the apparent damage, at least for the majority of people. Judging from people's behavior, most of them recover from the experience. Nevertheless, a significant minority of kids probably do carry their divorce-related problems with them when they leave home. Such problems may eventually interfere with their own efforts to form happy relationships and marriages.

THE IMPACT OF DIVORCE
ON THE NEXT GENERATION

The high rate of divorce in the United States in the 1970s and 1980s meant that several million children of divorce came of age in a short period of time around 1990. Psychologists and sociologists began studying this population, many of whom, they said, were showing ill effects.

A 1991 book, *Adult Children of Divorce* by Edward Beal and Gloria Hochman, reported: "An analysis of thirty-two studies, most of them conducted during the past fifteen years, reveals that adults of divorced parents have more problems and lower levels of well-being than adults whose parents stayed married. They are depressed more frequently, feel less satisfied with life, get less education, and have less prestigious jobs. Even their physical health is poorer." Throughout the 1990s, studies continued to appear in professional journals confirming these harmful effects.

Two widely read books published after 2000 challenged these findings, at least to a degree. Based on two different **longitudinal studies** (studies that follow a group of individuals over a long period of time), both books reported that many children survive and even thrive after their parents' divorces. They did confirm, however, that for a sizable minority of children, divorce caused problems that persisted for many years.

Fact Or Fiction?

Kids who have gone through a divorce do not
expect to ever be happily married.

Fact: Every major study has found that adult children of divorce believe in marriage as a goal for other people as well as for themselves. Even though they know firsthand the dangers and problems that marriage entails, most are willing to make the effort, and they are optimistic they will succeed. If anything, they are motivated to "rewrite their past," as one researcher put it, in order to provide a happier childhood for children of their own.

In the end, most children of divorce do get married themselves, often successfully.

In *The Unexpected Legacy of Divorce: A 25-Year Landmark Study*, psychologist Judith Wallerstein described her team's intensive personal interviews, at intervals of several years, with some 200 children from divorced families and from intact (nondivorced) families in the same neighborhoods. In summing up the findings, Wallerstein wrote, "Divorce is a cumulative experience. Its impact increases over time and rises to a crescendo in adulthood."

The majority of the children of divorce in Wallerstein's study had achieved somewhat more success in their working lives than the children of intact families (perhaps because divorce forced them to become more independent at an earlier age), and many were able to benefit from their parents' mistakes in building their own marriages. However, a significant minority of children of divorce did not do well in relationships. Thirty of the 93 children of divorce had never married, even 25 years after the divorce.

According to Wallerstein, many of the men were afraid of making commitments, due to a fear of rejection stemming from their parents' divorce. Many of the women had a pattern of casual and unsatisfactory relationships, and some married on impulse. They were sometimes unable to end a damaging relationship for fear of opening old wounds. The study found that even successful adults were often plagued with insecurity. They were afraid of conflict and change, and they could never shake off a sense that failure was always waiting around the corner.

Psychologist E. Mavis Hetherington's book *For Better or For Worse* was based on a less intensive but much larger survey. Hetherington came to more optimistic conclusions from her data, stating, "The big headline in my data is that *80 percent of children from divorced homes eventually are able to adapt to their new life and become reasonably well adjusted.*" Of her 900 subjects, 690 had married and only 189 of those who married had subsequently divorced. Even many of the adult children who felt that they had been "scarred" by their parents' divorce appeared to have successful relationships, as judged by the researchers.

The study did uncover a subgroup of some 20 percent who were "troubled" as young adults, with problems at work and in social relationships leading to poverty and divorce. Only 10 percent of the people in her study from intact families had similar issues. However, even this group showed less antisocial behavior with the passing years.

Hetherington's researchers devised a "marital instability scale" to measure components of good or bad marriages. They found that 36 percent of children of divorce had poor scores, compared with 29 percent of children from high-conflict intact families and only 18 percent of children from low-conflict intact families.

On the positive side, Hetherington found that most children of divorce remained close to their biological mothers, even when they were raised by their fathers. Only a third of the male children and a quarter of the females retained close ties with their fathers in their adult years.

RELATIONSHIP WITH DIVORCED PARENTS

When children from intact families leave home and begin to lead independent lives, they often come to see their parents in a different light. Faced with the difficulties of daily life, they can better appreciate what their parents managed to accomplish.

The same is true for children of divorce, who often had poor relationships with at least one parent during their childhood or teenage years. As they deal with their own financial and marital problems, they come to appreciate how difficult it must have been for their parents to deal with these issues along with the additional stress of divorce and, often, single parenting. Sometimes grandchildren provide an opportunity for reconciliation; sometimes the parents' lives have finally stabilized enough to rebuild ties with their children.

Reconciliation does not always take place. According to Wallerstein, "Elderly people with a history of divorce will get less care from their children than people who have never been divorced."

CHILDREN OF GRAY DIVORCE

The term *adult children of divorce* refers not only to those who were children when their parents divorced and have since grown up but also to those who were already adults when their parents split. While adults who may have families of their own can usually cope with their parents' divorce, the process can still have a disturbing emotional effect.

Divorce among older adults (sometimes called **gray divorce**) is relatively rare. The Census Bureau reported in 1990 that the divorce rate had remained steady since 1970 for married people over 65, in contrast to the huge increase in divorce among younger people. Only 10,000 men and 5,000 women over 65 get divorced each year. Nevertheless, these divorces can be a difficult event even for adult children, who often report that their happy childhood memories of family life "blew up in my face," as writer Noelle Fintushel reports in her book, *A Grief Out of Season: When Your Parents Divorce in Your Adult Years.*

These adults must build new relationships with each parent and between their parents and their own children. Some become alienated from one parent. They may be called upon to provide financial or practical assistance to one or both.

Of course, as today's generation of divorced people age, we can expect to see a higher and higher proportion of older Americans in

DID YOU KNOW?

More Older People Are Divorced

Even though few married people divorce once they are past age 65, there are more and more people that age and older in the United States who were previously divorced. The following table shows the percentage of men and women over 65 who are single, married, widowed, or divorced.

	Men				Women			
	1980	1990	1995	1999	1980	1990	1995	1999
Total (millions) of which (%)	9.9	12.3	13.2	13.7	14.2	17.2	18.5	18.7
Never married	4.9	4.2	4.2	3.6	5.9	4.9	4.2	4.0
Married	78.0	76.6	77.1	75.9	39.5	41.4	42.5	44.3
Widowed	13.5	14.2	13.5	14.0	51.2	48.6	47.3	44.9
Divorced	3.6	5.0	5.2	6.5	3.4	5.1	6.0	6.8

Source: U.S. Census Bureau, *Statistical Abstract of the United States*, 2000.

the divorced category. While the emotional and practical problems of the divorce may be in the distant past, this will still create some additional burden to society, since elderly people living alone (whether widowed, divorced, or never married) often require more assistance from family and society than those living with a partner.

Every major event in one's life leaves its effects. Divorce is one such event, for those getting the divorce and for their children. Most people get over the pain. The challenge is to learn the right lessons in order to build the best possible relations with all members of the divorced family and to avoid new divorces.

See also: Children, Psychological Effects of Divorce on

FURTHER READING

Ahrons, Constance R. *We're Still Family: What Grown Children Have to Say About Their Parents' Divorce.* New York: Harper Collins, 2004.

Fintushel, Noelle, and Nancy Hilliard. *A Grief Out of Season: When Your Parents Divorce in Your Adult Years.* Boston: Little, Brown and Co., 1991.

Hetherington, E. Mavis, and John Kelley. *For Better or For Worse: Divorce Reconsidered.* New York: W. W. Norton, 2002.

Wallerstein, Judith S., Julia M. Lewis, and Sandra Blakeslee. *The Unexpected Legacy of Divorce: A 25-Year Landmark Study.* New York: Hyperion, 2000.

■ HELP FOR TROUBLED MARRIAGES

Aid is available for unhappy couples who may be willing to stay married if they can resolve certain conflicts. Much of this book focuses on the negative effects of divorce. Some couples who may be fully aware of these negatives still decide to divorce, convinced that their unhappy marriage cannot be saved. Other unhappy couples are willing to stay married, if they can find a way to resolve certain conflicts or resentments. They may still have positive feelings for one another or common interests that could form the basis of a renewed relationship. Some couples may be willing to put up with a less-than-perfect marriage for a period of time to spare their children economic or emotional problems.

Where can such people turn for help? Ever since the divorce rate began to soar in the 1970s, hundreds of books have been written on the subject for those who are willing and able to begin the work on their own. A sympathetic ear from an impartial adviser is usually helpful too. In cities and towns across the nation, thousands of counselors, therapists, and public and private agencies have developed programs and techniques in recent years to help people avoid divorce.

COUNSELING

The methods for helping people save their marriages go under many different names: counseling, therapy, coaching, marriage education, mediation, and no doubt others. The goals are usually similar. Most try to keep couples focused on current problems and needs rather than analyze how the problems arose. They help people find practical solutions for the future.

Some of these goals include:

- Identifying and helping to satisfy each person's individual needs as well as the couple's relationship needs
- Uncovering hidden agendas
- Working to reduce negative ways of relating to each other
- Encouraging positive activities the couple can do together

Personal needs

Even the most caring, unselfish person has needs. These may include love, respect, power and control, success at work, sexual gratification, financial security, a beautiful or comfortable home, hobbies, friendships—the list can go on and on. People with too many unsatisfied needs may feel depressed, worthless, or irritable. They may devote too much attention to the few areas where they can find satisfaction, resulting in overwork, overeating, or some form of addictive behavior. Any of these reactions is dangerous for a marriage.

Husbands and wives may have somewhat different or even conflicting needs. But couples who can voice these needs have a better chance of dealing with the inevitable frustrations.

Uncovering the hidden agendas

If couples tend to fight over small issues, chances are **hidden agendas** are at play. Hidden agendas are issues or problems that are not discussed openly but can attach themselves to any topic of discussion in unpredictable and often destructive ways. For example, some spouses feel that their partners do not appreciate their contributions or respect their opinions. If the partner disagrees with something as minor as the choice of movie to rent, it can cause a major fight.

According to the popular self-help book, *Fighting for Your Marriage* (written by family therapists Howard Markman, Scott Stanley, and Susan J. Blumberg), four common types of behavior may be signs of hidden issues:

- Wheel spinning; arguments are repeated with no progress toward resolution

- Trivial triggers; minor matters cause major fights

- Avoidance; one or both partners postpones or deflects discussions on important matters

- Scorekeeping; one or both partners insists "I'm always the one who..." or "You're always doing..."

Even when hidden issues are brought to the surface, they are usually hard to discuss—that's probably why they were hidden in the first place. People may be embarrassed to admit feelings of inadequacy, need for control, or sexual frustrations, but it's worth the effort to try, given the alternatives. If the issue turns out to be a marriage-breaker, a divorce might well have taken place anyway, but at the cost of even more confusion and animosity.

Healthier patterns of relating

Couples can fall into bad habits in their relationships without being aware of them. Sometimes it takes an outsider—a sensitive counselor or therapist—to see patterns of behavior that people in a relationship cannot see by themselves.

Bad habits can include consistently failing to hear what the other spouse is saying, refusing to discuss important topics when they are raised, and putting negative interpretations on innocent or neutral remarks. A marriage can survive such behaviors, but even if it does, it can become a demoralizing experience for both spouses.

Build up the positives

A couple may successfully deal with some hidden or unmet individual needs, learn better ways of relating, and still not feel motivated to continue the marriage. Eliminating the negative is only one side of the equation; accentuating the positive is the other side. Fortunately, that side can be easier and less stressful to accomplish.

A couple that has been devoting time and effort toward working through problems might want to dedicate some of that time to discussing the things that keep them together. Love, respect, and gratitude should not be taken for granted.

Busy parents, in particular, often find they do not spend much time together. Many have little energy after work, parenting, and chores to just have fun with each other. The good times that brought them together in the first place no longer seem to happen. They probably won't happen, unless both partners make a deliberate effort to set aside time alone together on a periodic basis. Some couples may deliberately devote more time and energy to their children's needs, but the kids certainly do not benefit if the parents' relationship gradually weakens or if too few positives remain to outweigh the inevitable negatives.

FAMILY SUPPORT

Family support programs provide result-oriented help to families suffering from a range of problems, including troubled marriages. Begun in the 1970s, these programs rely on resources from multiple government and private agencies to help families anticipate, prevent, and overcome problems.

Some of the organized groups that promote the concept of family support also lobby government agencies, legislatures, and large employers in support of proposals they believe will help families stay together. Many large institutions, including the military, have instituted family support programs, on the theory that family problems interfere with productivity and cause higher employee turnover.

SUPPORT GROUPS IN THE COMMUNITY

Other support groups in many communities are dedicated to keeping marriages together by directly addressing husband-wife issues and conflicts. Many of them focus on education *before* marriage. For example, churches and religious organizations have united in a few hundred American towns to create **community marriage policies** (CMPs), which encourage premarital educational programs and provide assistance to troubled marriages. The engaged encounter program sponsored by the Roman Catholic Church offers premarital counseling to people not only in the United States but also in many other countries.

There are no magic solutions to most marriage problems. Even marriages that have been repaired can come apart again as a result of new pressures. But few goals are more worthy of hard work than saving and improving a marriage that might otherwise slide down the road to divorce.

See also: Divorce Alternatives; Love and Marriage; Stress Factors in Marriage, External

FURTHER READING
Markman, Howard J., Scott M. Stanley, and Susan L. Blumberg. *Fighting for Your Marriage.* San Francisco, CA: Jossey-Bass, 2001.
Mordechai Gottman, John, and Nan Silver. *The Seven Principles for Making Marriage Work.* New York: Crown, 1999.

■ LOVE AND MARRIAGE

Most Americans believe that love and marriage are inseparable; as the song says, they "go together like a horse and carriage." Who, however, has a horse and carriage anymore?

A CBS poll taken in 2001 found that 64 percent of married Americans and 43 percent of unmarried Americans believe that romance never goes out of a marriage. This is not a universal view; some cultures regard marriage less romantically; they see it as a legal, social, or financial arrangement that may or may not involve love. Are those cultures more realistic than ours?

Fact Or Fiction?

Romantic love is a recent invention in Western culture. In the old days, people didn't "fall in love."

Fact: Not true. Every civilization seems to have some concept of romantic love. It is found in the Bible and in the literatures of ancient Egypt, Mesopotamia, China, India, and Japan. People in preliterate societies have described feelings of love to visiting anthropologists.

On the other hand, love has not always played the central role in marriage that it does today in the United States. In many cultures, it is common for families to arrange marriages on behalf of their children. In some cultures, men are then allowed to pursue love outside of marriage; women are usually not granted that privilege.

No one can deny the power of love to make people overcome their own selfish instincts. In today's stressful world, many marriages would not survive if husband and wife did not draw strength from their love to overcome problems. Of course, love can take many forms—mad infatuation, "best friends," "comfortable old shoe," love-hate sparring match. The same couple can pass through more than one phase, and back again, in the course of a long marriage.

Should every couple who falls in love seek to get married? These days, many of them decide to cohabit rather than marry. A few controversial experts, such as Dr. William Pinsof of Northwestern University, recommend that society adopt a new standard for pair bonding that would make **cohabitation** and **co-parenting** (where mother and father live apart but share in raising their children) as acceptable as marriage.

For people who do get married when they fall in love, if that love fades, should the marriage end as well? Can people maintain a healthy marriage and family without some form of love? Can a couple maintain a healthy marriage if only one partner is still in love?

STAYING TOGETHER FOR THE SAKE OF THE KIDS

Most people would find divorce a reasonable choice for a loveless marriage as long as no children were involved, but what if young children or teenagers are in the picture? Given the complications of divorce and the emotional pain it usually brings to kids, should responsible people endure a loveless marriage "for the sake of the kids"?

Many people advise couples to do just that. As long as there is no open animosity or conflict, they say, parents should grin and bear it for their children's sake.

People who consider themselves practical and unromantic often point to arranged marriages, which are common in many parts of the world. In Japan, the divorce rate for arranged marriages is lower than for "love marriages." Should parents in loveless marriages take heart from that example and avoid divorce? Would that be unfair to themselves? Consider what kind of life they may have if they follow that advice.

TEENS SPEAK

Arranged Marriage? Great, but Not for Me.

Raya is a 12-year-old Iranian-American girl who came to the United States as a baby with her parents and teenage sister. Her sister got married a few months later.

"It was totally an arranged marriage," Raya explains. "Before we came to America, she was sort of engaged to Shorosh, even though they had never met in person. She had a chance to say no, after they spoke on the telephone and wrote a couple of letters. But he seemed okay to her, so she went ahead."

According to Raya, her sister's marriage is successful. Both sets of parents helped the couple at the beginning, buying them a condo and then babysitting while the young couple worked.

"My sister says she loves her husband, but I don't always believe her. Whatever, it's not for me. America isn't Iran. First of all, any guy in America who lets his parents find him a wife is not for me. Who wants to spend their life with someone they don't love? What if I meet someone afterward and I totally fall for him? What a mess, huh?"

Luckily for Raya, her parents understand her feelings, and say they would never even try to arrange a match for her.

One possible path is an **open marriage,** in which the partners are free to have relationships with other men or women, either platonic (without sex) or not. Aside from moral and religious objections, most parents—especially mothers—with more than one child would laugh at the suggestion. When would they have the time? In any case, such an arrangement might be more upsetting to the children than a divorce.

Some parents in a loveless marriage may be capable of postponing their hopes for romantic love until their children are older. Love for their children and other family members and friendships at work and in their community can go a long way toward filling that empty space in the heart. After all, divorce is no guarantee that a new, loving relationship will come to either partner.

MARRIAGE VOWS

Wedding vows used to be fairly standard in the United States. The exact wording may have varied among religious groups, and justices of the peace may have added their own personal turns of phrase, but the principle was the same.

Before witnesses and in the presence of a higher authority (God, or a representative of the state), the bride and groom made a series of sacred promises to each other (or accepted the promises as recited by a religious leader or judge). They agreed to be loving and faithful partners and help each other through good times and bad. Most couples pledged to remain married "as long as we both shall live," or "till death do us part." Often the bride promised to obey her new husband, and the groom promised to support his new wife, in keeping with certain religious beliefs about gender roles.

These days, many brides and grooms write their own vows to better reflect their personal values and goals. Many books have been written providing sample vows to help these couples, and many wedding Web sites do the same. Often they leave out wording that implies different roles and responsibilities for husband and wife, and sometimes they leave out the pledge to remain together for life.

An Internet search early in 2004 of popular wedding Web sites that included prewritten vows found 40 vows that included a pledge to remain together for life and 31 vows that did not. People may be adjusting their expectations of marriage to conform to today's experience.

Without exception, all the prewritten vows stressed love as the crucial pledge. People seem to be promising to love one another for as long as they remained married. If they fail to fulfill that part of the vow, are they still obligated to honor the other pledges—support, respect, and companionship?

In the end, everyone has to make his or her own decisions. Whether one decides to get married or divorced, love is usually a crucial part of the calculation. However, since love is both irrational and powerful, it makes sense that people consider their choices carefully before committing themselves to the responsibilities of marriage or deciding to end that marriage, solely based on the promptings of their hearts.

See also: Divorce Alternatives; Marriage Lifestyles, Alternative; Relationships, Types of

FURTHER READING

Lee Smith, Susan. *Wedding Vows: Beyond Love, Honor, and Cherish.* New York: Warner Books, 2001.

Roney, Carley. *The Knot Guide to Wedding Vows.* New York: Broadway Books, 2000.

■ MARRIAGE COUNSELING

See: Help for Troubled Marriages

■ MARRIAGE LIFESTYLES, ALTERNATIVE

Ways in which some couples share their lives outside the bounds of traditional marriage.

Most people think of divorce as an option only for legally married couples. However, millions of Americans now **cohabit** (live together as couples without being married), or are **domestic partners** (two people who are recognized by an employer or a municipality as a couple for the purpose of employee and other benefits). These couples often raise children together, sometimes in jointly owned homes. Like married couples, they often break up too, and experience similar problems and issues.

Until recently, nearly everyone in the United States assumed the institution of marriage applied only to **heterosexual** couples (one man/one woman). However, in recent years male and female same-sex couples are trying to win marriage rights too. They have made gains in a few states and Canadian provinces and in several European countries, although they have also met vocal opposition in much of the United States.

The Census Bureau reported that the 2000 census counted some 600,000 **gay** (same-sex) couples, about equally divided between man/man and woman/woman. These couples share many of the characteristics of married people.

TRADITIONAL MARRIAGES

Millions of households in the United States are still built on the old-fashioned model of the **nuclear family**, defined as a husband, wife, and their biological children living together in their own home. Census Bureau figures indicate that this type of arrangement is not headed for extinction.

Fact Or Fiction?

The traditional family as we know it in America is dead.

Fact: The U.S. Census Bureau reported in April 2001 that the number of children living in nuclear families rose between 1991 and 1996, reversing a declining trend that had apparently been in effect for about 20 years.

The Bureau defines a nuclear family as a married couple living together with their biological children. In 1996, 56 percent of all American children were living in such families, as compared with 51 percent just six years earlier. An additional 15 percent of kids were living in other types of two-parent households in 1996.

Researchers attributed the trend to a decline in divorces and a leveling off of births out of wedlock.

Many of these nuclear families have stay-at-home mothers. In 1998, 42 percent of children under six years old living in married families had a stay-at-home parent (usually the mother), as did 32 percent of kids ages six and seven, according to the Department of Health and Human Services. Of course, in 1960, 82 percent of women with kids under six stayed at home.

MARRIAGE AMONG WORKING COUPLES

The new model of the American family, in which the woman works outside the home and the man participates more directly in raising kids, has had a major impact on divorce. Before the 1970s, divorced mothers in the United States nearly always got custody of their children, because they were seen as the child-care expert and the "nurturing" spouse. Men typically won limited visitation rights, which usually did not include overnight stays.

Today's courts are more likely to award custody to fathers, although mothers are still the primary care givers. Divorce mediator Joan B. Kelly estimated in 2003 that fathers received **sole physical custody** of their kids (the children live with them all the time) in about 15 percent of divorces in the 1990s, up from about 10 percent in the 1970s and 1980s.

DOMESTIC PARTNERSHIPS

Until recently, couples who cohabited had none of the legal rights or responsibilities of married couples. Only in a few states could a man and woman who lived together be recognized as having a **common-law marriage** if they stayed together for a certain number of years. By the 1980s that situation had begun to change, thanks to a new status called domestic partnership.

About 200 cities, counties, and states in the United States now have laws allowing unmarried couples of the same or opposite sex to register as domestic partners. These couples must provide evidence that they live together and share some financial responsibilities. In addition to providing some of the benefits of marriage—such as hospital visitation rights—these laws generally provide formal procedures for ending the partnership, the equivalent of divorce.

A growing number of public and private companies and organizations provide employee benefits to the domestic partners of their employees. These benefits are equivalent to those provided to married couples. According to the advocacy group Human Rights Campaign in 2004, some companies extend these benefits only to same-sex domestic partners, arguing that opposite-sex partners have the option of legal marriage. Many clubs and cultural organizations offer family memberships to same-sex partners as well.

Q & A

Question: How many employers offer health benefits to domestic partners of their employees?

Answer: According to the Human Rights Campaign, in January 2004 over 7,200 employers offered benefits to domestic partners of their employees, including:

- 212 of the Fortune 500 companies
- 6,655 smaller firms and nonprofit organizations

- 10 state governments (California, Connecticut, Iowa, Maine, New Mexico, New York, Oregon, Rhode Island, Vermont, and Washington)

- 130 city and county governments (including Atlanta, Baltimore, Chicago, Denver, Los Angeles, Milwaukee, Minneapolis, New Orleans, New York, Phoenix, Pittsburgh, San Diego, San Francisco, Seattle, and Washington, D.C.)

- 198 colleges and universities

SAME-SEX FAMILIES

Contemporary historians such as John Boswell in his 1995 book *Same-sex Unions in Premodern Europe*, have found evidence that some gay people (those sexually and emotionally attracted to their own sex) lived together as couples in every historical era. Some of these relationships lasted a lifetime, with couples owning homes, supporting one another, and even raising children.

In the past, those children were usually the product of earlier marriages to people of the opposite sex. Today many are adopted, and others are the biological child of one of the partners, using donated sperm or surrogate mothers.

Historians do not know how many such gay couples existed at earlier times. The government and religious bodies that recorded marriages and divorces would have considered the topic unmentionable. In fact, until the twentieth century many people were uninformed about homosexuality as a way of life.

Until recently, few gay couples acknowledged their status openly, for fear of losing their jobs, being evicted from their homes, or being physically attacked. In some cases, they maintained separate residences even while living together most of the time.

Since the 1970s the taboo has largely disappeared. Gay couples have found more and more acceptance from neighbors and society as a whole. Some are willing to declare their status publicly.

Some gay couples have sought religious marriage ceremonies. A handful of individual clergy from each of the major faiths have been willing to preside over such ceremonies. A few associations of churches and synagogues have also approved ceremonies for gay couples, though they are usually not considered full weddings. The

DID YOU KNOW?

Unmarried Partners, Same and Opposite Sex

	Number (millions)	Percent
Households	105	100.0
Coupled households	60	56.9
Unmarried partners	5.5	9.1
Opposite-sex unmarried partners	0.6	8.1
Same-sex unmarried partners	0.6	1.0
Male partners	0.3	0.5
Female partners	0.3	0.5

Source: U.S. Census Bureau, 2000.

Metropolitan Community Church, an association of several hundred gay-oriented Protestant churches, performs over 6,000 same-sex weddings a year.

Starting in the 1990s, gay couples in several states sued for the right to marry, while gay advocacy organizations petitioned state legislatures to include gay couples under marriage laws.

In 2000, as a result of a decision by a state court, Vermont became the first state in the United States to implement a form of legal marriage for same-sex couples, known as a **civil union**. In the first two years, nearly 5,000 couples (two-thirds female) were granted civil unions in Vermont; about 90 percent were from other states. Between 2000 and 2002, only 10 of these couples dissolved their union.

While the Vermont case was making its way through the courts, courts in Hawaii were debating the same issue. In light of the publicity surrounding such cases, Congress overwhelmingly approved the Defense of Marriage Act in 1996, which was then signed by President Bill Clinton. The law declared that the federal government would not recognize same-sex couples as being married. It also allowed any state to refuse to recognize a same-sex marriage issued by another state.

In 2003, following Canada's decision to allow same-sex marriages, some Americans called for a constitutional amendment to prohibit states from doing the same. The movement attracted additional support in November 2003, when the Massachusetts Supreme Judicial Court ordered the state legislature to make provisions for same-sex marriage in that state beginning in May 2004.

TEENS SPEAK

My Other Mom

"Everybody thinks it's funny—gay people getting married—but to me it's very serious."

Dylan has always had a mother and a father. They are his biological parents, who divorced when he was still a toddler. He doesn't see much of his dad, who lives in another state, but they speak twice a month and he receives presents and money in the mail. When he was seven years old, he got a third parent, his mother's partner, Anita.

"Anita is really the one who takes care of me the most. My mom works long hours in her store. Anita is the one who cooks and cleans, because she only works part time. And her parents are way cool, the best."

Dylan has only told one friend about his family situation, but other kids sometimes guess, and sometimes give him a hard time.

"I don't care. To me, Anita is just as much my parent as Mom. I think I'm luckier than some of my friends who live with just their mother. I don't see why Mom and Anita aren't allowed to get married. It isn't fair, in my opinion."

Dylan, who is 14, doesn't have a girlfriend, but he hangs with a bunch of guys and girls from school.

"When I ever want to bring home a girl, I want her to know that I believe in getting married. And I want her to see that that's the kind of family I have, even though it doesn't look that way from the outside."

See also: Custody and Visitation; Relationships, Types of

FURTHER READING
Coleman, Marilyn, and Larry Ganong, eds. *Points and Counterpoints: Controversial Relationship and Family Issues in the 21st Century.* Los Angeles, CA: Roxbury Publishing Co., 2003.
Moats, David. *Civil Wars: A Battle for Gay Marriage.* Orlando, FL: Harcourt, 2004.

■ MEDIA AND DIVORCE

The topic of divorce as treated in literature, the arts, and the mass media (the newspapers, television, and other outlets that aim to reach most of the public); the relationship between the media and public opinion.

From the 1940s through the 1960s, movies and television shows in the United States generally avoided the subject of divorce or the difficult issues surrounding it. The print media—newspapers, magazines, and books—were more willing to tackle the subject, but they often used a sensationalistic, gossipy tone.

The media reflected the public's general view of divorce, tending to disapprove except in cases of abuse or adultery. In fact, in literature and film many divorce stories ended with the unhappy couple reunited in love and marriage, unlike most unhappy couples in real life.

Two trends that came together around 1970 dramatically changed this view of divorce. Popular attitudes about divorce rapidly changed, as Americans started getting divorced in numbers never seen before. At the same time, the media became much freer in their treatment of many controversial issues, including divorce.

As a result, divorce became far more visible, with numerous movies, books, and TV dramas treating the subject. Even situation comedies featured divorced characters. Divorce was not only visible; it was increasingly portrayed in a positive light, as a reasonable option for some married people.

By the 1990s, film, TV, and book critics began debating the subject of "divorce in the media." Reporters, college professors, and counselors who worked with parents and children disagreed as to whether the media were presenting divorces fairly. Some even argued that the media was part of the problem; they said it painted too positive a picture of divorce and ignored the downsides. Others insisted that the media had the opposite bias, emphasizing the negative side of divorce in order to promote old-fashioned values. Still other writers believed that the media were simply reflecting the complicated lives and values of ordinary people in all their variety and confusion.

In other words, divorce has become part of the **culture wars**. This term refers to the many controversies over values among different groups in the United States. Disagreements on topics such as divorce, single and unmarried parenting, the role of religion in the nation, sexual behavior, abortion, pornography, and substance abuse have come to play a large role not only in the political arena but also in education and the entertainment industry.

PORTRAYALS IN LITERATURE

Critic Barbara Dafoe Whitehead's influential and controversial 1996 book, *The Divorce Culture,* is often used as a starting point for debates about the influence of the media on marriage and divorce. According to Whitehead, the literature of divorce has gone through several phases in the United States.

In the late 19th and early 20th centuries, prominent novelists like Henry James and Edith Wharton were willing to tackle the subject of divorce, and they did not avert their eyes from some of its harmful effects. Wharton sometimes showed divorce as a tool that women could use to assert their independence; strong women in her novels used marriage and divorce as paths to financial security and power. According to Whitehead, Wharton was also blunt in showing the downside of divorce on a couple's children.

This stress on the impact of divorce on children was also evident in the widely popular etiquette books of the first half of the twentieth century. Authors like Emily Post saw divorce as a necessary evil; she argued that divorced people should be accepted and treated with respect and discretion, largely to limit conflict and protect their children.

John Cheever's 1950 story "The Season of Divorce" helped reintroduce the subject to serious literature, according to Caitlin Shetterly, editor of a 2001 book of divorce stories called *Fault Lines.* However, the subject did not become a major topic until the 1970s. According to Whitehead and other critics, most of the flood of books in the "first wave" of divorce literature in that decade looked at divorce as an opportunity for personal growth on the part of ex-spouses.

Books aimed at men sometimes encouraged divorced men to exploit their new sexual and romantic freedom without guilt or shame. The larger number of books written for women saw divorce

as part of a journey of emotional growth. Some books even specu-
lated that children would benefit from divorce, because they would
be spared the conflict of unhappy marriages and their parents would
be happier.

Books written for children since the 1970s have often been more
realistic. The counselors and therapists who wrote or inspired these
books stressed that children of divorce need to learn that they are not
alone; other kids are going through the same difficult process. In any
case, kids who have gone through divorce would probably not be
interested in books that sugarcoat their experience.

Via its Web site, the American Academy of Pediatrics advises writers to give "an accurate depiction of how children feel and behave
when parents divorce." Writers are encouraged to study the guidelines
given to divorcing parents about how to handle their children.

Whitehead claims that classic children's literature (prior to recent
decades) typically stressed the role of parents as rule-givers and caretakers. In contrast, some of the recent divorce books for kids have
reversed traditional roles. They ask kids to understand their parents'
problems and to help them through the difficulties of divorce.

PORTRAYALS ON TV AND IN MOVIES

In the early 1900s, the American motion picture industry was rather
freewheeling and uninhibited. Without rules and formats to guide
them, the many small companies and studios of the time turned out
pictures of different types to appeal to a new, diverse audience. Sex,
violence, and immoral behaviors found their way into the movies, in
part as a reflection of the new urban lifestyles and values of the
1920s, in part as a way to sell as many tickets as possible.

By 1934, however, public opinion, as expressed by many city governments and the influential Catholic Legion of Decency (an organization of Roman Catholic clergy and lay people that sought to
suppress what they saw as immoral and harmful behavior) forced the
industry to censor itself. Under the "Hays Code" (named after its cre-
ator, Will Hays) no movie was allowed to threaten "the sanctity of the
institution of marriage and home." Divorce could be portrayed "only
for sound reasons, as a last resort, and never lightly or flippantly." In
the economic hard times of the 1930s, sobriety and responsibility
seemed more important to many people than individual freedom.

For the next 30 years, relatively few films dealt with the topic,
according to lawyer-historian Michael Asimow in his study, "Divorce in

the Movies." Those films that did present divorce frequently ended with reconciliation (such as *The Women* in 1939). If the film did not end in reconciliation, at least one party was always clearly at fault, and he or she suffered greatly after the divorce (as did the unfaithful wife in Sinclair Lewis's novel *Dodsworth,* which was made into a film in 1936).

The Hays Code was abandoned by 1968. According to Asimow, the first major American film to seriously deal with divorce and its issues was the 1979 drama *Kramer vs. Kramer.* Feminists were among those who claimed that the movie portrayed the unhappy wife and mother as the villain of the story. However, even critics agreed that the film revealed the emotional trauma of divorce and raised issues about custody battles and the difficult economic effects of divorce. These issues have continued to appear in countless movies since.

Television has followed a similar path, with divorce and divorced characters becoming more and more present in the broadcast schedule. Whitehead claims that while such programming may help children deal with the pain of divorce, these shows also "carry an unmistakable message about the impermanence and unreliability of family bonds."

Fact Or Fiction?

In the "old days," American movies did not tackle controversial subjects like divorce.

Fact: Not true. Before the "Hays Code" was adopted by the movie industry in 1934, films about divorce were fairly commonplace. According to the American Film Institute, 171 such films were made in 1911–20, and 182 films in the following decade. The pace actually doubled in the period 1931–34, when an average of 34 films about divorce were made each year. From 1935 to 1940 the number fell to 21 per year, and it declined even more to 11 per year in the 1940s.

As long as divorce remains a common feature in American life, it will be covered in the media, for better or worse. Whatever approach the media takes, the public—individual readers or viewers—will decide for themselves which books and shows help them understand the phenomenon and deal with its impact.

See also: Divorce in America

FURTHER READING

Leibman, Nina C. *Living Room Lectures: The Fifties Family in Film and Television.* Austin, TX: University of Texas Press, 1995.

Parish, James. *The Hollywood Book of Love.* New York: McGraw-Hill Contemporary Books, 2003.

Whitehead, Barbara Dafoe. *The Divorce Culture: Rethinking Our Commitments to Marriage and Family.* New York: Vintage Books, 1996.

■ MONOGAMY

See: Relationships, Types of

■ RACIALLY AND CULTURALLY MIXED MARRIAGES

Marriages between people who were born into different ethnic, racial, or religious groups.

Until a 1967 Supreme Court ruling, many states had **antimiscegenation** laws (laws against racial mixing), which made it illegal for people of different races to marry, live together, or have sexual relations. Even in the other states, many people disapproved of marriages across racial or religious lines.

Since that ruling, the United States has become a more tolerant multicultural country. Mixed marriages of all kinds have become more common, and many people adopt children of races other than their own. Immigration from all parts of the world makes it likely that racially and culturally mixed marriage will increase in the years to come.

In fact, even the meaning of the word *race* has changed. A hundred years ago most people thought that the common racial categories (black, white, yellow, red, and brown) were based on biology. People now understand that those racial categories have almost no scientific standing, but are merely popular notions based on ignorance. According to biologists, there are greater differences between individuals who are considered to be in the same race than between those of different races.

Mixed marriages have become commonplace. Mixed couples are raising a generation of several million mixed-race children. The number of mixed marriages between people of different religions and ethnic groups (groups with a common national or cultural origin) seems to be increasing as well in the United States, as immigrants continue to assimilate into the wider culture.

Q & A

Question: How many interracial marriages are there in the United States?

Answer: According to U.S. Census Bureau estimates released in 2003, about 3 percent of all married couples in the U.S. in 2002 were racially mixed. That amounts to nearly 1.7 million couples, or over 3 million people.

The numbers have been increasing dramatically. Between 1970 and the present, the number has quintupled. Over 90 percent of those couples have one white partner, with the other partner coming from every other racial group in the country. Marriages between the other racial groups have been increasing as well.

Couples who **cohabit** (live together) are even more likely to come from mixed backgrounds. According to the Center for Family and Demographic Research at Bowling Green State University, 13 percent of couples who were cohabiting in 1998 were of mixed racial background, as compared with 5 percent of married couples who were racially mixed.

A study of 1990 U.S. Census data compiled by the University of Michigan Institute for Social Research in 2000 found that one out of eight black men who cohabited did so with a white woman; while only 25 percent of married Asian women had white husbands, 45 percent of cohabiting Asian women had white partners.

RACIALLY MIXED FAMILIES

Interracial couples have a slightly higher divorce rate than same-race couples, according to statistics from the National Center for Health Statistics in 2002. Forty percent of same-race couples divorce after 15 years, compared with 47 percent of mixed-race couples. The data suggests that racial differences may be a significant stress factor in mixed-race marriages, though one quite possible to overcome. Despite wider acceptance, mixed couples and families still meet with hostility on occasion, causing practical and emotional problems.

Whatever differences a married couple may have, as long as they are from a similar racial background, those differences may be invisible to the outside world. Racially mixed families do not have that luxury. Their differences are more likely to register, at least as a matter of curiosity if not hostility, with neighbors, strangers, and their children's friends. Even a rare overheard remark by a foolish or disturbed individual can be hurtful and frightening to children. In addition, each partner in a mixed marriage is likely to hear occasional racist remarks about his or her partner's race from people who don't know about the marriage.

While people who marry outside their race may be tolerant and curious of other traditions and communities, their relatives are not necessarily so open-minded. Racism from one or both sides, family memories of past persecution, and individual acts of discrimination mean that even couples who are not personally affected by racism may be affected indirectly through relatives.

Marriage expert Dr. Keith Whitfield reports in his 2001 book *Fighting for Your African American Marriage* that black and other minority same-race couples can internalize stress imposed on them from racial slights and mistreatment and then redirect their anger at each other. Interracial couples, he writes, may respond to similar pressures in an even more destructive way: One spouse may come to use the other as a symbol of his or her race.

To complicate matters further, few individuals are completely free of the legacy of prejudice and intergroup animosity. However, with honesty, humility, and of course love, couples can work through these problems, as many of them are happy to testify.

Up until a generation ago, a child with one white and one nonwhite parent was generally classified by society as belonging to a nonwhite race. Today most people consider children born to a mixed-race couple as mixed-race; since the 2000 census, the U.S. Census Bureau allows people to identify themselves as belonging to more than one race.

Mixed-race children may choose to identify with either or both of their parents' races as they grow up. In addition, many same-race couples are now adopting children of another race. At least 10,000 foreign babies and children are adopted by U.S. parents each year, many of them of a different race than their new parents. The number of interracial adoptions within the United States has begun to rise as well, following the passage of a federal law in 1994 making it illegal to deny placement of a child solely on the grounds of race or national origin.

TEENS SPEAK

Who Isn't Mixed?

It wasn't until Sundar's family moved to a different state that he ever thought of himself as anything but an American kid.

"In Palo Alto there were so many kids from all over the world. The kids from India especially looked up to me as this real sweet American dude. In Wyoming it was different, maybe because of my name or maybe because Dad's skin is so dark. I have a Hindu name, but to be honest I don't really know much about the Hindu religion.

"I came home crying the first day; these kids were just yanking my chain, but I was only nine and I took it seriously. I didn't want to go back to school. Then it got even worse, because my parents started fighting about it. This sounds funny, but I never even used to think of them as mixed-race before we moved. I mean, who isn't mixed? Every race is a mixture anyway. People can't even guess what my background is—sometimes they think I'm Latino."

Over time, the situation improved. Sundar's parents eventually joined the church to which several of his school friends belong; they are active in the food bank and other programs.

"The funny thing is, my father is teaching me more about my Indian heritage too, at the same time that he plans to be baptized. Whatever works, is what I say."

CULTURALLY AND RELIGIOUSLY MIXED FAMILIES

Many of the pressures on interracial couples come from outside the home. In contrast, unique problems relating to life within the family often arise in marriages that are **interreligious** (spouses from different religious backgrounds) or intercultural (spouses from different ethnic backgrounds).

The Census Bureau does not collect statistics on people's religion, but many religious and ethnic organizations have done their own research. They consistently report that marriage between people of different religious and cultural backgrounds has become common-place in the United States.

About 30 percent of all U.S. marriages sanctioned by the Catholic Church in 1997 were interfaith, according to the Catholic magazine *Commonweal* in 1998. A study by the Council of Jewish Federations starting in 1990 claimed that over a third of American Jews married outside their faith. In recent decades, 64 percent of marriages taking place within the Greek Orthodox Archdiocese of America involved a bride or groom from another faith. An article in the *Journal of Marriage and Family* in 2002 found that 80 percent of Arabs born in the United States (whether Christian or Muslim) had non-Arab spouses. Muslim, Hindu, and Buddhist groups have also reported rising inter-marriage, especially among American-born children of immigrants.

The impact of these marriages may be complicated. For many years, studies have consistently found higher rates of troubled mar-riage and divorce among interreligious couples. For example, an arti-cle by Professors Evelyn Lehrer and Carmel Chiswick in the journal *Demography* in 1993, based on a sample of more than 3,000 couples, found that "religious compatibility between spouses at the time of marriage has a large influence on marital stability."

Young couples in love cannot always predict how strong their reli-gious beliefs or ethnic ties may become over time. These beliefs and ties become clearer as a couple approaches crucial milestones like buying a home, having children, choosing their children's education, or even meeting their children's friends or dates. Different expectations about gender roles and ties with relatives can cause problems from the start, as can practical issues like which holidays to celebrate and how.

In some families, differences of opinion about religious issues may fade with time, particularly if one spouse becomes active in the other's religious community through a formal conversion. However, other couples have managed to build stable marriages despite contin-uing differences on this subject, sometimes with the help of support groups composed of similar couples or after reading the growing number of self-help books on the topic.

Mixed marriages of all kinds may well be the wave of the future in the United States. The increased scale and variety of immigration, the growth of higher education and travel, and the globalization of culture—all are bringing together people from different backgrounds. People being what they are, some will fall in love and marry, thus ensuring that mixed families will become more and more common.

See also: Religion and Divorce

FURTHER READING
Crohn, Joel. *Mixed Matches: How to Create Successful Interracial, Interethnic, and Interfaith Relationships.* New York: Fawcett Columbine, 1995.
Grapes, Bryan J., ed. *Interracial Relationships.* San Diego, CA: Greenhaven Press, 2000.
Romano, Renee Christine. *Race Mixing: Black-White Marriage in Postwar America.* Cambridge, MA: Harvard University Press, 2002.

■ RELATIONSHIPS AFTER DIVORCE, PARENTS'

Divorce professionals often say, "a divorced family is still a family." That seems almost obvious when the cast of characters remains the same after the divorce as before: two parents—who now live apart—and their kids. Families become more complicated, however, when new players enter the picture.

Either of the parents—or both—may have a new partner at the time of the divorce; in fact, that relationship may have been the main cause of the divorce. If not, there's a good chance both parents will eventually find other partners, whether for occasional dates, a live-in relationship, or a second marriage. These partners, in turn, may have children of their own from a previous marriage. Is this still a family?

Clearly, the family has changed. Even when all of the original family members are still in contact with one another and frequently interact, their relationships are different. They will change even more as new partners and siblings enter the picture.

These changes may be difficult and painful, and each family member will react in his or her own unique way. Some may benefit from new arrangements, others may be indifferent, and still others may feel threatened and hurt as they lose some of the attention and support they have taken for granted.

Children can be in any of these categories. Even when things work out to their benefit, they usually have to deal with uncomfortable emotions. They probably have to learn new ways of relating to each parent, which can be a tall order for kids who have their own growing-up problems to deal with.

JEALOUSY: EX-SPOUSES, CHILDREN

Most couples who divorce are still emotionally involved with each other, sometimes for years. Even when they agree to separate, one or both may still love his or her ex-partner, particularly if only one of the two wanted the divorce.

Those divorced couples who cannot have a simple conversation without anger and hostility are also involved with each other, but in a different, more negative way. When a new girlfriend or boyfriend appears, emotions can become explosive.

Jealousy is a basic human feeling that anyone who has been in love has probably experienced. Divorced people may be particularly vulnerable, especially the partner who is still alone. Jealousy can be irrational; even the spouse who has already found a new partner may feel jealous when his or her ex-spouse finds a romantic interest as well.

Most divorced people understand that when a former spouse becomes involved with another person, they must swallow their pride and move on. However, they are not always able to hide their feelings from their children. They should try; as psychologist Florence Bienenfeld wrote in her 1995 book, *Helping Your Child Through Your Divorce,* "It is unwise to saddle a child with having to protect a 'wounded' parent."

Children can be jealous too. As a rule, they do not like competition for the attention and affection of their parents. Older kids in intact families often resent new babies; they are even more likely to resent a new baby who comes to the family through remarriage.

A **custodial parent** (the one the kids live with) often has particularly close ties with his or her children. As long as the custodial parent remains single, his or her life often revolves around the kids. When a new date shows up one Saturday evening, a child may see the newcomer as a threat to a close relationship with the parent.

Q & A

Question: If my divorced mother starts dating, how will she still have time for me and my siblings?

Answer: Chances are your mother shares your concerns. But after all, even married parents go out once in a while, and they still have time for their children.

You may really fear that your mother may not have enough *love* for you. Try to discuss your feelings with her. If you don't share your fears, how will your mother know about them, much less respond to them?

Younger children may not hesitate to ask, "Will you still love me if you fall in love with_____?" Older children may phrase the question in a more roundabout way, but both have every right to ask. Many parents raise the topic themselves. Some children can become so jealous that they try to compete with their parent for the new friend's attention.

CHILDREN'S RELATIONSHIP WITH PARENTS

Jealousy may be only one of the issues that arise for children when their divorced parent has a new relationship. It may not even be the most important.

Perhaps the first reaction of many kids is disappointment. No matter how clearly parents have explained that the divorce is final, their children may still secretly hope the parents will get back together. Children who feel this way are likely to become angry with the dating parent and anyone he or she dates. The anger will be difficult for everyone concerned, but it may actually help some kids face the reality that their parents' marriage is over, especially if a year or two has gone by.

Children may react to a parent's dating by being protective of the other parent. A certain amount of concern is a sign of love and thoughtfulness. However, it is usually best for the other parent to deal with the issue without involving the kids.

If the new relationship becomes serious, some children may start to worry that the new adult in the family may change their mother's or father's parenting style, especially if the friend seems to be stricter than the parent. Parents need to be aware of these concerns and talk them over with their kids as clearly as they can.

Some kids are embarrassed that their parent is dating, which they think of as a teenage behavior pattern. They also may think their parents are acting inappropriately when they try to improve their appearance or behave more youthfully. Kids can be inappropriate at times too, by trying to act as their parent's chaperone or protector.

Children's discomfort with a parent's dating behavior can sometimes be treated with humor on both sides—kids can tell their father, "Act your age," and he can reply, "Don't be a geek." However, a parent's sexual behavior can be a more serious matter for kids. Experts advise divorced parents to be discreet about their sex life. Divorce expert Judith Wallerstein reported in her 2000 book *The Unexpected Legacy of Divorce* that young girls in her study who were exposed to casual sex between a divorced parent and other adults were likely to become promiscuous at an early age, with serious consequences for their health and emotional stability. Boys often reacted by abusing alcohol and drugs.

CHILDREN'S RELATIONSHIPS WITH PARENTS' SIGNIFICANT OTHERS

Children may eventually accept or reject a parent's new **significant other** (friend, lover, or spouse) on the basis of their individual qualities and behavior. The process, however, can take years.

Younger children may find it easier to accept the new person from the start. As a rule they tend to accept anyone who is friendly and open. Adolescents (those between 12 and 20) are more likely to compare the new friend with the other parent, which may not be fair to the friend. After all, who can compare with a child's own mother or father?

TEENS SPEAK

"We Didn't Like Her at All"

Things went from bad to worse for 14-year-old Christopher and his younger sister, Sara. They were just getting used to living in two places (two weekends a month with Dad, the rest of the time with Mom), when their father told them his girlfriend, Melissa, was moving in.

"We didn't like her at all," Christopher later said. "I still think she's just after his money. That's what my mother says too."

At first Christopher refused to go to his dad's as long as Melissa was there, but after a while he gave in. "They made my sister go, and I didn't want to leave her alone over there. It's not like I'm angry with Dad, but I think he's making a big mistake.

"I told him so, right to his face. He took us to a hockey game last time we were there, and we had a long talk. He asked me to give Melissa a chance. He said that if we still didn't get along, he'd work something out."

Christopher isn't sure he believes his father, but he does admit that in some ways things have gotten better since Melissa moved in.

"He used to be out on dates every Friday night and sometimes Saturday night too. At least now he stays home with us. But I wish my parents would stop changing my life around. It's not fair, we're only kids."

One way for a new friend to ruin his or her chances with a partner's children is to interfere in their discipline. Even a stepparent is usually unsuccessful in imposing authority on stepchildren, but a live-in lover will almost never succeed. Children may believe the new person is trying to replace the other parent, especially if he or she criticizes or demeans the other parent.

Children should understand that it is unlikely that they will change their parents' mind about a new friend; on the other hand, they certainly have a right to express their feelings. A wise parent will respect these feelings, and try to work the problem out as much as possible.

Sometimes the opposite problem occurs. Children develop an emotional attachment to the parent's new friend before the parent is sure the relationship will last. The last thing a child of divorce needs is the loss of another close adult.

Divorced parents may sometimes prefer **cohabitation** (living together) with their new partner instead of marriage, in case the relationship does not last. They may not realize that children can be just as upset by the breakup of such a relationship as they are to a divorce.

On the other hand, some kids are happy when their parents find a new partner. A happier parent can sometimes be more relaxed and more attentive to his or her children.

A parent's new friend can become a friend to the kids as well—someone to help with homework, organize fishing trips, or put some order into the home (which some single parents find difficult to do on their own). Kids may feel guilty that they are betraying the other parent if they show affection to the newcomer. But they can still show both parents love and support when they are together. The situation calls for consideration and respect all around.

Fact Or Fiction?

If a boyfriend or girlfriend moves in with a custodial parent, the court can take the children away from that parent.

Fact: While this was often true in the past, it is very unlikely to happen today. In fact, live-in lovers don't even affect child support payments in most cases. Since the new partner has no obligation to help support the children, the biological parents are still expected to honor the agreement currently in force. Even if the custodial parent remarries, most courts will not reduce the noncustodial parent's child support payments.

However, when a same-sex partner moves in, judges in many states will agree to reopen a custody agreement, and children are sometimes removed from the home of the gay parent.

See also: Divorce, The Psychological Cost to Spouses of; Families, Blended

FURTHER READING

Ellison, Sheila. *The Courage to Love Again: Creating Happy, Healthy Relationships after Divorce.* San Francisco, CA: HarperSanFrancisco, 2002.

McKay, Matthew, Peter Rogers, Joan Blades, et al. *The Divorce Book: A Practical and Compassionate Guide.* Oakland, CA: New Harbinger, 1999.

■ RELATIONSHIP FAILURE

The problems that can arise *within* a marriage, when husbands and wives relate to each other in unhealthy or destructive ways.

What makes so many marriages succeed? Love, companionship, common interests and goals, and a sense of responsibility toward children are all crucial factors. Plenty of stamina and plain old grit are also indispensable—plus the patience to muddle through. Unfortunately, a marriage can fail for many reasons too. The list of potential challenges includes:

- External problems that couples have no control over but still must handle in some way, such as serious illness, death in the family, or job loss
- Internal problems that result from the character or personality of one or both partners, such as addictive behavior, inability to compromise, or a tendency toward avoidance and distance
- Physical or sexual violence
- Infidelity
- Falling out of love

LIFE CHALLENGES AND STRESSES
Most new marriages start off on a wave of optimism. Good thing, too. Unless they're very lucky, most couples can expect to face problems as time goes by that would upset even the most confident people.

Many serious problems are caused by events beyond the couple's control, such as a job loss or chronic illness. Special needs children as well as aging parents can make huge demands on a couple's physical and emotional resources while draining their morale. Even normal life-cycle events, such as a child going away to college or a parent reaching a milestone birthday, can have unpredictable effects even on marriages that were models of success up until that point.

DYSFUNCTIONAL FAMILIES: CODEPENDENCY, CONFLICT, EMOTIONAL DISTANCE
The term **dysfunctional family** has been used so loosely on TV talk shows and in magazines that almost every family can be called "dysfunctional." But relatively few truly deserve that description. Properly speaking, the term refers to families that tolerate physical, emotional, or sexual abuse; those with one or both parents unable to carry out their role due to illness or substance abuse; or those with parents and children unable to relate to one another in a consistent, caring way.

Some destructive behaviors, such as violence and abuse, are relatively easy to detect. Others are less obvious but also quite harmful—such as codependency or emotional distance.

The life of a **codependent** individual is organized completely around the needs and feelings of another family member (or other close person). Of course family members should help and support one another, but codependents go overboard. Their excessive behavior is often harmful not only to themselves but also to the interests of the spouse or parent they are trying to help.

The term was first used to describe those spouses or children of alcoholics who unintentionally supported their loved one's alcohol dependency. Psychologists eventually observed the same unhealthy behavior pattern among people reacting to any type of addictive behavior in a loved one. According to the National Mental Health Association Web site, codependency can be passed from one generation to another. A husband or wife who grew up in a codependent family may later repeat the pattern of excessive self-sacrifice in his or her own marriage, even if the spouse is not addicted.

A codependent often tries to control the spouse through overprotection. The excessive attention and care leaves little time for the codependent's own needs; he or she may then blame the spouse for ruining his or her life. Codependents sometimes enable their spouses, that is, make excuses for bad or addictive behavior rather than help to overcome it.

In the end, codependency leaves both partners unsatisfied and often leads to divorce. Ironically, when an alcoholic sobers up, the codependent spouse is sometimes unable to adjust to a newly healthy partner.

Another destructive behavior pattern is persistent conflict between spouses, when every disagreement becomes a win-or-lose fight. Arguments or fights are not always bad. On the contrary, couples should face their differences honestly, even at the risk of a verbal spat. An occasional argument can serve to relieve tension; a couple that makes up after an argument may find their relationship stronger than before.

When arguments or shouting matches seem to take place all the time, however, the marriage is clearly in trouble. Psychologists, such as Susan M. Jekielek in a 1998 article in the journal *Social Forces,* warn that a high-conflict home environment can be damaging to children. Unfortunately, if a couple does not learn how to head off or control conflict, even divorce may not solve the problem; it only adds new sources of disagreement—financial support, child custody, and new relationships.

Therapists and counselors have developed techniques that can help two people handle disagreements better, including the following ones.

- If a difficult issue needs to be discussed, choose the time of day that is the least stressful and leave enough time for a reasonable conversation.
- Repeat each other's points to prevent misunderstanding and to show each partner is listening.
- Focus on the issues, not the personalities.
- Don't dredge up old issues. Complain about a behavior only when it happens—not after the fact.
- Call time-outs to collect thoughts and overcome anger.

Even if the disagreements cannot be resolved and divorce is inevitable, the whole family is better off if parents can learn some of these techniques.

Ironically, couples who *never* argue may be facing another problem—emotional distance, or withdrawal, where one partner is "not there" emotionally for the other. When a quietly dying marriage reaches the point of divorce, it usually comes as a shock to the children in the family. Children do not usually pay as much attention to silence as to conflict.

Everyone in a family does not have to be equally talkative. People have different styles, sometimes based on family or cultural traditions. For example, in some cultures a good father and husband is the "strong silent type" who shows his love and concern through actions rather than words. However, if a couple needs to address important problems, they may need to seek help from counselors who can "draw out" the silent partner.

VIOLENCE IN MARRIAGE

Domestic violence (violence between family members, also called **intimate partner violence (IPV)** to include cohabiting and dating couples), is a widespread problem in most countries, including the United States. Every year thousands of women and a smaller number of men (who represent 5 to 15 percent of victims, according to the Centers for Disease Control and Prevention), are killed or maimed as a result of domestic violence.

Fact Or Fiction?

Men are always the abusers in domestic violence; women are always the victims.

Fact: Even though men can be victims too, women are far more likely to be seriously injured or killed by criminal violence on the part of their partners than men are to be hurt by their partners. According to the Justice Department's National Crime Victimization Survey, in 1998, 160,000 men were the victims of a violent crime by an intimate partner, as compared with 876,000 women that same year. In both cases, the figures included some same-sex violence.

Violence leading to serious injury occurs in nearly 5 percent of American couples, according to a 1996 article published by the National Institutes of Mental Health. Violence affects families from every religious and ethnic group and at every economic level. Not even pregnant women are immune—some 350,000 are attacked by their partners each year, according to the National Center for Injury Prevention and Control.

Violence is unacceptable and must be opposed by the full force of the law. Following increased public attention and concern over the past few decades, some progress has been made. According to Department of Justice statistics, between 1993 and 2001, the number of violent crimes by intimate partners against women dropped from 1.1 million to 590,000; against men, the numbers dropped from 163,000 to 103,000.

Some couples may be able to overcome occasional violence by learning conflict-management techniques. However, an ongoing pattern of violence is difficult to treat, and separation is often the only solution. Ironically, the process of separation and divorce can provoke more violence. Researcher Judith Wallerstein reported in her 2000 book, *The Unexpected Legacy of Divorce,* that while a quarter of the husbands had been violent toward their wives in the years leading up to divorce, fully *half* became violent in the period of the divorce itself.

Thousands of women have survived only by fleeing with their children to shelters for battered women (women routinely abused by their partner). From the relative safety of such shelters, they can seek out police intervention and court-issued **protection orders**, which require the abusive partner to keep away from the spouse or children.

DID YOU KNOW?

Intimate Partner Violence (IPV) in Georgia

This table shows the percentage of women in each category who reported such violence.

Category	Percent who reported violence
Age	
15–24	7
25–34	6
35–44	3
Education	
Less than high school	11
High school graduate	5
Some college	4
College graduate	2
Living arrangement	
Married	3
Separated	21
Divorced	12
Widowed	0
Cohabiting	9
Never married	6

Source: Centers for Disease Control and Prevention; Georgia Public Health Department, 1998.

Wallerstein and other researchers report that daughters in particular suffer severe emotional effects when their fathers are violent toward their mothers. A girl's sense of self-worth may suffer, and she may herself become more vulnerable to abusive relationships. Nevertheless, in most states family courts will grant a violent spouse visitation rights with his or her children following divorce, as long as no violence has been directed at the children themselves. In extreme cases, courts may assign a neutral adult to participate in these visits.

Unfortunately, many women in such couples are afflicted with **battered woman syndrome**—a pattern of behavior in which a woman accepts the violence without resistance, sometimes even denying that it is taking place. Such women may feel guilty and inadequate because they have not been able to protect themselves or their children.

Today, even the most determined opponents of divorce usually encourage spouses to leave violent relationships. Divorce is often painful for kids—but not nearly as disturbing as an atmosphere of violence and profound insecurity.

TEENS SPEAK

It's Just Too Scary

Stephanie and Emily are both quiet, slim, and short for their age—14 and 15, respectively. But don't be fooled by their fragile appearance.

"Once we had to get between our parents, physically, to push them apart when they were fighting, and I mean *push*. It was like being a wrestling referee on TV."

Stephanie still looks frightened as she speaks.

"It was getting to where they would fight every day. Ma always had bruises on her face and all over her arms, black and blue marks. We never called the police, because we were afraid they would take Emily and me away. A couple of times I did pick up the phone to call 911; but then I wussed out."

Their parents are in the process of divorcing. In the meantime the girls are living with their mother, though they see their father about one week each month.

"They never touched us," Stephanie insists as her sister nods. "Honestly, neither of them even yelled at us. It was just each other. They're both hot-blooded, and I guess they got off on the wrong foot a long time ago. They go together to a marriage counselor now, but truth? I hope they can be friends again, but they should keep apart. It's just too scary any other way."

RAPE IN MARRIAGE

Until the late 1970s, most states did not consider it a crime for a husband to rape his wife (forcing her to engage in sex). While some state laws still show vestiges of this attitude, in general state and federal laws have come into line with common sense and humanity. No man has a right to force his wife, partner, or date to comply with his sexual desires.

The message has taken a long time to get through to a significant minority of men. According to a 1994 Department of Justice report, husbands, former husbands, boyfriends, and ex-boyfriends commit 26 percent of all rapes and sexual assaults.

As with intimate partner violence in general, there are several risk factors that increase the danger of spousal rape. These include:

- Alcohol or drug use
- Male partner's unemployment
- Either partner witnessing domestic violence as a child, or being beaten as a child
- Poor communication skills
- Depression and low self-esteem

INFIDELITY

The "old-fashioned" idea that husbands and wives should be faithful toward one another has never gone out of style. In fact, it has grown stronger in recent years, according to the National Opinion Research Center at the University of Chicago. Surveys the Center conducted in the 1990s found that between 78 and 80 percent of Americans believe adultery is "always wrong," compared with 70 to 72 percent who felt that way in the 1970s.

Q & A

Question: How common is adultery?

Answer: Not as common as people think, according to the National Opinion Research Center (NORC) at the University of Chicago. In five separate surveys between 1991 and 1998, people participating in NORC's General Social Survey were asked the following question: "Have you ever had sexual intercourse with someone other than with your spouse when you were married?" Only 12 percent of women and 21.5 percent of men answered yes. The question was asked on a private questionnaire, and NORC's sociologists believe the results are close to the truth.

Mutual trust is essential for married people. It is unreasonable to expect a spouse to accept without complaint all the work and sacrifice that marriage and parenthood impose, when a straying partner is ignoring his or her need for love, respect, and support.

In 1972 sociologists Nena and George O'Neill caused a sensation with their book, *Open Marriage*. They claimed that affairs with other people could strengthen a marriage. They said that the demand for sexual fidelity (remaining faithful to a single partner) was a leftover from the days when women were considered the property of their husbands. Within a decade, the couple had publically retracted their views. Today no respected psychologist or sociologist downplays the importance of fidelity in a relationship.

FALLING OUT OF LOVE

Today, many women are able to earn a good living on their own and being single is no longer viewed as a shameful status. Therefore couples are more likely to separate and divorce when they fall out of love. In particular, people who are financially secure and do not need their spouse's income to survive seem to be more likely to pursue their right to love and happiness.

The challenge for parents is to reconcile their own needs with those of their children. Parents may feel that a loveless marriage is not the best environment to raise children, but few psychologists agree. They maintain that children typically assume that their parents are in love until confronted by conflict and separation.

Singer Paul Simon's 1973 single "50 Ways to Leave a Lover" struck a chord in many listeners. It is not hard to end a relationship; saving one is much harder. However, anyone who wants to find and keep a partner in life eventually must learn how it is done.

See also: Help for Troubled Marriages; Stress Factors in Marriage, External

FURTHER READING
Biggers, Jeff. *Chemical Dependency and the Dysfunctional Family.* New York: Rosen Publishing Group, 1998.

Jenkins, Pamela J. and Barbara Parmer Davidson. *Stopping Domestic Violence: How a Community Can Prevent Spousal Abuse.* New York: Kluwer Academic/Plenum, 2001.

Presma, Frances and Paula Edelson. *Straight Talk about Today's Families.* New York: Facts on File, 1999.

■ RELATIONSHIPS, TYPES OF

Not every adult in an intimate long-term relationship is married. Couples can date, live together, or be involved in nonexclusive relationships. Any one of these situations can end in a breakup, with results that can look very much like divorce.

MONOGAMY

Most people still believe that the ideal lifestyle is **monogamy**, in which both parties to a marriage or relationship refrain from sexual or romantic relations with anyone else. The full weight of the moral and religious heritage of most Americans supports monogamy, which implies love, loyalty, mutual support, and stability—just the qualities children need the most from their parents.

However, the word *monogamy* has more than one meaning. The Merriam-Webster Online Dictionary lists three definitions: 1) the practice of marrying only once during a lifetime; 2) the state or custom of being married to one person at a time; and 3) the condition or practice of having a single mate during a period of time.

The dictionary labels the first definition (once in a lifetime) as out of date. Nevertheless, millions of Americans do in fact stay married for life, and most of the rest keep looking for a life partner. The Catholic Church continues to regard marriage for life as the only acceptable ideal.

The second definition is the most commonly used today—one marriage at a time. A lot of people these days have been married two or more times, but they are still practicing monogamy in this sense. They get divorced before each new wedding. People who get married a second time without divorcing their first spouse are practicing **bigamy**, which is against the law throughout the United States and Canada. A small number of Mormons and a handful of others illegally practice **polygamy**, in which a man has more than one wife at the same time.

The third definition of monogamy, having a single "mate" at a time, not necessarily in marriage, describes a large and growing population of cohabiting couples (people who live together without get-

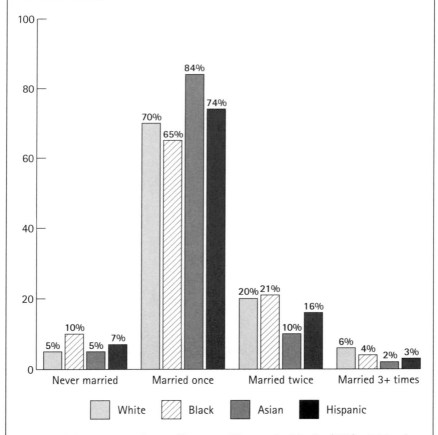

DID YOU KNOW?

Number of Times Married

This chart counts only people age 45 or older, as younger people have had less time to marry twice, not to mention three or more times.

Source: U.S. Census Bureau, Survey of Income and Program Participation (SIPP), 1996 Panel, Household Economic Studies, February 2002.

ting married). If they are faithful to each other and give each other mutual support, many people would call them monogamous. Some adults who are in long-term dating relationships—they regularly keep company but do not live with their partner—may also lay claim to being monogamous. However, no one would use the term *monogamy* to describe long-term **open relationships,** in which people have a primary partner but continue to date others.

SERIAL MONOGAMY
AND MULTIPLE DIVORCES

Even when divorce was rare in the United States, there were social circles in which it was widespread. Popular newspapers and magazines throughout the 20th century gave wide coverage to the romantic lives of movie stars and wealthy people, some of whom would change husbands and wives as often as some teenagers change boyfriends and girlfriends.

In the 1960s, sociologists came up with a term for this phenomenon—**serial monogamy.** They probably did not expect it to become as common as it has. The numbers are hard to pin down, but according to a 2002 Census Bureau report, 22 percent of those in their forties had been married two or more times by the age of 40. Nevertheless, the Bureau could still say, "Most adults have married only once."

Serial monogamy may actually be declining. The Centers for Disease Control and Prevention (CDC) reported in 2002 that while 65 percent of women who divorced in the 1950s later remarried, the percentage had fallen to 50 percent for women who divorced in the 1980s. However, if cohabiting couples are considered "monogamous," serial cohabitation would have to be included in the statistics for "serial monogamy."

Whatever the exact numbers, the impact on families in the United States may be substantial, especially among children. E. Mavis Hetherington, a divorce expert, reports that in her study, "Serious emotional or behavior problems were found in only 20 percent of children whose parents had gone through a single divorce, but in 38 percent of those coping with multiple divorces." Judith Wallerstein, another expert who has often warned of the harm of divorce to children, reports that due to remarriage, breakups of cohabitations, and serial dating relationships, "Most children of divorce experience not one but many more losses."

TEENS SPEAK

They Could Make a Team

Lots of kids have a stepfather. Maxwell has had two, and he's not sure he's seen the last of them.

"It's a good thing I don't have sisters. I can't see my dad taking care of any girls, so they'd have to live with Mom all the time, and it would probably drive them crazy.

"My dad is a slob and my brother and me have to sleep in the living room; plus, he hardly ever gives us any money. But at least at his place there's peace and quiet. I love my mom, but I get real angry if I stay with her for too long, and I start yelling at her."

Max's parents got divorced seven years ago, when he was six years old. His mother remarried after a couple of years. "She wanted to give us a big house, summer vacations, but it didn't work out. My stepfather had money but he used to drink and carry on; he even hit me a few times. So Mom had to throw him out, and they got divorced too. Then she found Bill. He's OK, for a stepfather, but he travels a lot on business, and Ma's getting real tired of that. She told me last week she can't take it any more, but I said if she divorces him too I'll never stay with her again. I don't know if I mean it, but I sure don't plan to live with another stepfather."

COHABITATION

For millions of American adults, **cohabitation**, or "living together," has replaced marriage as the preferred relationship, at least for a certain period in their lives. Census Bureau figures show a huge increase in recent decades in the number of **POSSLQs**, which is the bureau's term for unrelated, adult "persons of the opposite sex sharing living quarters."

The bureau assumes that these individuals are cohabiting. Only 523,000 POSSLQs showed up in the 1970 census; over 5 *million* were counted in 2000. In fact, the CDC tells us, fully half of all 30-year-old women have cohabited at some time in their life.

Many people cohabit to see if they are compatible enough to marry. In fact, 70 percent of couples who cohabit for more than five years eventually marry, according to a 2002 study by the Center for Family and Demographic Research at Bowling Green State University. Other people may avoid marriage because their families oppose their choice of a mate. A 1998 survey by the same center found that cohabiting women were more likely than married women to be older or better educated than their partners. The center also found more than twice as many interracial and interethnic cohabiting couples as married couples.

Sociologists give many explanations for the growth in cohabiting, which shows, if nothing else, that the social stigma that used to prevent these arrangements has all but disappeared. Some economists have

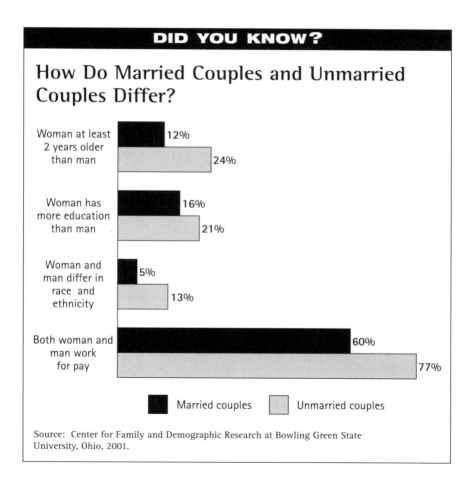

DID YOU KNOW?

How Do Married Couples and Unmarried Couples Differ?

Woman at least 2 years older than man: 12% (Married) / 24% (Unmarried)

Woman has more education than man: 16% (Married) / 21% (Unmarried)

Woman and man differ in race and ethnicity: 5% (Married) / 13% (Unmarried)

Both woman and man work for pay: 60% (Married) / 77% (Unmarried)

■ Married couples   ▢ Unmarried couples

Source: Center for Family and Demographic Research at Bowling Green State University, Ohio, 2001.

explained the decline in marriage and the increase in cohabitation in terms of the theory of "rational choice," which predicts that people will govern their life choices based on economic costs and benefits.

According to these scholars, women who generally plan to remain in the workforce whether they marry or not and who expect to earn about as much as their partners, have less incentive to marry than women in previous generations. Also, since divorce has become so commonplace, and divorce as a rule no longer provides for **alimony** payments, women cannot assume (as they once could) that marriage will provide them with greater financial security than simply living together does.

Many cohabiting couples have children living with them—43 percent by 1998, according to the Center for Family and Demographic Research study, as compared with less than 30 percent in 1978. Government and private agencies studying divorce are paying increasing attention to cohabiting families in order to get a more comprehensive view of parenting and divorce.

Q & A

Question: How many kids live in unmarried families?

Answer: The U.S. Census Bureau reported in 2002 that over 3 million children under the age of 18 were living with one parent and that parent's unmarried partner. That figure represented between 4 and 5 percent of all kids.

The National Institute of Child Health and Human Development reports that 40 percent of all children will live in a cohabiting family for at least some period of time before they turn 16.

In addition to the 11 percent of kids who are born to cohabiting parents (who may be their biological parents, and who may later get married), 20 percent of children born to married parents will eventually live in a cohabiting household after their parents' divorce. Finally, more than three-quarters of kids born to a single parent will see that parent move in with an unmarried partner.

DATING

When two adults say they are dating each other, they usually mean to imply an exclusive relationship. While they may have different residences, they spend time together periodically, perhaps some of it at each other's homes.

On the other hand, when divorced people say they have "begun dating," they may simply mean they now have the time and emotional strength to go out with potential partners. Many books on divorce contain advice to people who may not have dated for years or decades, explaining the changes in customs and reminding readers of the common-sense rules of social interaction.

Unlike teens, adults who date are usually looking for a stable, long-term relationship. In a majority of cases, the relationship either ends or leads to cohabitation or marriage.

OPEN RELATIONSHIPS

In what is known as an open relationship, either partner is free to date other people. People can set rules as they please; they may agree to be honest with each other about their dating activities, or they may decide to be discreet and not mention other dates. They may agree to allow only one-time or casual encounters, or to leave all options "open." Dating may be allowed, but not sex—or just the other way around.

"Open relationships" are usually more acceptable to one partner than the other, who may go along only until a more satisfying option appears. Open relationships often lead to jealousy, hurt feelings, and resentment, as one partner is more likely to expect or feel more than the other.

Fact Or Fiction?

If two adults are mature, experienced, and honest with each other, they can have a satisfying long-term "open relationship."

Fact: Not true. Experts, therapists, and advice columnists from nearly every point of view agree that it is very unlikely for a man and a woman to build a stable long-term relationship if they are unwilling or unable to accept some level of exclusive commitment.

If one partner is not hurt when the other one dates, chances are that he or she may just not care about the relationship. Anyone looking for love and a steady partner would be smart to find someone who wants that too.

In the course of adult life the average person today has several different intimate relationships, usually a combination of single or multiple marriages, cohabitations, and dating. As a consequence, people often go through several breakups, each one potentially as complicated as a divorce. Each breakup also can affect any children still living at home.

See also: Divorce Alternatives

FURTHER READING
Paul, Pamela. *The Starter Marriage and the Future of Matrimony.* New York: Villard, 2002.
Warner, Ralph, Toni Ihara, and Frederick Hertz. *Living Together: A Legal Guide for Unmarried Couples.* Berkeley, CA: Nolo Press, 2003.

■ RELIGION AND DIVORCE

Religion plays a major role in the life of many Americans. In fact, the United States is known as a religious country. What impact does that religion have on marriage and divorce?

Most Americans identify with one of the three major monotheistic religions: Christianity, Judaism, and Islam. In all three, the clergy—priests, ministers, rabbis, and imams—used to perform all marriages and divorces according to their own laws and customs without interference from the government. Even today some 75 percent of U.S. marriages take place in houses of worship, according to the Massachusetts Child Support Enforcement agency.

Divorce is common even among adherents of religious denominations that officially frown on the practice. Furthermore, most religions are divided into different denominations, each of which has its own interpretations of traditional laws. In addition, recent immigration from Asia has brought new religious communities to the United States, such as Buddhists and Hindus.

Q & A

Question: Do Native American religions allow married couples to divorce?

Answer: Many Native American tribes in what is now the United States seem to have allowed married couples to separate. Among some, the custom was for one of the two divorcing partners to leave the local community. Typically it was the husband who left or was told to leave—a wife could announce divorce simply by placing her husband's belongings outside the door. The children remained with the partner who stayed put. The home and domestic property remained in the woman's possession, while the man kept any horses, cattle, or crafts he had made himself.

All religions place a strong emphasis on marriage and family, although some are more tolerant of divorce than others. In a 2000–2001 survey by the Barna Research Institute, the divorce rate (which averaged 34 percent for all adults) was 33 percent among those who called themselves "born again" Christians, 32 percent among Protestants in general, 30 percent among Jews, 29 percent among Catholics, and 24 percent among Mormons.

Most religious groups consider widespread divorce to be a serious problem. In response, many Protestant ministers and Catholic priests in nearly 200 American towns and cities have joined to create **community marriage** policies (CMPs). These clergy agree that couples marrying in their churches have to participate in premarital counseling and workshops, often with married couples serving as "mentors." They also have to observe a waiting period of at least several months before the wedding can take place.

INTERFAITH MARRIAGE AND DIVORCE

Many Americans marry outside their own faith; the number of **interfaith marriages** seems to be increasing. About 50 percent of all Jews, 40 percent of Muslims, and about 35 percent of Roman Catholics in the United States marry outside their faith, according to the *Christian Science Monitor* in 1997.

When interfaith marriages end in divorce, the parents often disagree on their children's religious practice after divorce. They may come to an agreement only in the divorce settlement, or a solution may be imposed by a judge.

Most courts try to enforce the *status quo*, the family's practice before the divorce. If the children were raised in a particular faith or attended a specific church, judges may instruct the parent not to have the child formally converted to another religion.

In some cases, judges have told parents to refrain from exposing their children to religious environments that demean or condemn the religion they were raised in before the divorce, since that might cause "actual or substantial harm." However, balancing the best interests of children with each parent's religious beliefs can be difficult.

TEENS SPEAK

Between Two Faiths

Henry's parents are in the middle of a messy divorce. He understands that they are fighting over custody and religion, among other things, but they won't tell him the details. "They tell us we're not old enough. I'm actually 14 already, but I have two younger brothers that are only seven and nine. I know that my father is not Catholic anymore, and my mother is *very* religious."

Henry says his father joined a Pentecostal church just a few months ago. He took the boys there once; when his mother found out, she was very angry. "I didn't like it so much anyway because it wasn't Catholic, and that's what we were brought up on—the priests, and the candles, and all the pictures. It always makes me feel so peaceful, every Sunday.

"And the pastor can't even speak English. But my father used to do drugs and he says the new church is the only thing that keeps him straight, so I hope he keeps going."

Whatever the lawyers and the judges decide, Henry hopes they make up their minds soon, and let things settle down. "I'm old enough to make up my own mind anyway about God and things. As long as nobody forces me, I think I will manage OK."

PROTESTANTS AND DIVORCE

Among Christians throughout the world, the various Protestant denominations have historically been more tolerant of divorce than Roman Catholics and Eastern Orthodox. In the United States, most Protestant denominations accept divorce as a necessary evil. Protestant ministers and clergy usually allow divorced people to remarry in church.

Each denomination, and sometimes each congregation, has different rules and practices regarding divorce. The United Church of Christ and the Unitarian Universalists have developed specific rituals for divorce. Episcopalians used to require a dispensation from a priest or bishop to get remarried, in keeping with the old traditions of the Church of England. Today, all but a few traditionalist churches in the denomination allow divorced people to remarry in church.

Some Baptist churches oppose divorce except on grounds of adultery; ministers will not remarry the partner who committed adultery and may bar him or her from leadership positions. On the other hand, many Baptist churches have special ministries to divorced persons, recognizing how common divorce has become.

CATHOLICS AND DIVORCE

The Roman Catholic Church considers marriage to be a sacrament or spiritual act before God that cannot be undone. Therefore, the church does not recognize divorce and does not permit divorced Catholics to remarry.

According to the Philadelphia Archdiocese, "The Catholic Church cannot end or break a valid marriage bond between two baptized persons." Any Catholic who divorces and remarries is considered to be guilty of adultery and is not allowed to participate fully in church rites.

Fact Or Fiction?

In the Catholic Church, anyone who gets a divorce is excommunicated—he or she cannot receive communion or other holy rites.

Fact: A civil divorce does not affect a person's religious status according to the Roman Catholic Church. Both partners are still considered to be in a valid marriage, and thus can receive communion. The problem arises when a divorced person remarries without getting a Catholic annulment. That person is then considered to be an adulterer and is generally not allowed to receive communion.

On the other hand, the Catholic Church sometimes gives a married couple an **annulment**, which is a statement that the marriage was not valid to begin with. When one partner petitions for an annulment, a church tribunal (court) tries to determine whether both of the partners were of sound mind and body at the time of the wedding and whether they understood the responsibilities of a Catholic husband and wife. The other partner has a right to be heard, but his or her agreement is not necessary.

For example, the tribunal might determine that the husband or wife never intended to have children and therefore had not entered the marriage in good faith. In that case, the marriage was not valid, and the tribunal annuls it. They may even annul a non-Catholic wedding, if one of the partners now wants to marry a Catholic. After the annulment, the two partners are free to remarry, provided they get a civil divorce.

In recent years, public opinion polls have found that a large majority of Catholics disagree with the church's position on divorce. While Church leaders have so far refused to change policies, they have greatly increased the number of annulments, from just a few hundred a year in the 1960s to tens of thousands a year in the 1990s and 2000s.

JEWS AND DIVORCE

Jews regard marriage as a contract between a man and a woman, each of whom has specific rights and responsibilities. Either partner can seek a divorce if the contract has not been honored (for example, if one partner withholds financial support or lives apart). Divorce can also be granted on grounds of incompatibility.

The two parties in a divorce negotiate financial and custody terms. A rabbinical court of three rabbis can resolve any differences, with each party represented by its own rabbi. After the divorce both parties are allowed to remarry.

According to traditional Jewish law, the husband issues the divorce decree, but generally needs his wife's approval. If a wife refuses, a husband can still divorce her on certain grounds, but only with the approval of 100 rabbis. A woman cannot get divorced if her husband does not agree, although rabbis occasionally issue annulments or decree that a missing husband is deceased.

In recent years, organizations have arisen among Orthodox Jews (those who interpret traditional law strictly) that pressure husbands to divorce wives they have abandoned. Many Orthodox rabbis insist that grooms agree in writing before the wedding that they will pay heavy penalties if they leave their wife without a divorce.

Only about 15 percent of American Jews are Orthodox. The Conservative movement in Judaism also requires that people obtain a religious divorce before remarrying, but Conservative rabbis are more likely to invalidate a marriage at the wife's request. Reform rabbis usually accept a civil divorce decree as the equivalent of a religious one.

MUSLIMS AND DIVORCE

Islam, the religion of Muslims, has always permitted divorce. Muhammad, the founder of the religion, spoke out against the practice, but he did allow it in some cases. Over time Muslim law has codified the grounds for divorce and the various procedures for obtaining one.

- A husband and wife can decide to end a marriage by mutual consent without the involvement of a Muslim court of law. Often the wife returns the **dowry** (payment from the groom's family) that she received at the marriage, especially if she is the one who wants the divorce.

- Traditionally, a Muslim man has the right to divorce his wife by saying *talak* (divorce) three times. He must then abstain from marital relations for four months for the divorce to be valid. A woman can have the same right, but only if it was written into the marriage contract. Generally, the husband must compensate his former wife financially, if she does not have independent means.

- Either husband or wife can petition a Muslim judge for a divorce. Women usually take this approach. Grounds for divorce can include failure to fulfill marital responsibilities, impotence, or leaving the Muslim faith.

The Muslim community in the United States is relatively new, and Muslim courts and judges often are not available, although some local imams (religious officials or scholars) can help Muslim couples draw up the appropriate documents. Many American Muslims are married to non-Muslims. As a result, many of these couples avoid the religious process and only obtain a civil divorce. The rate of divorce seems to have gone up among Muslims in the United States, according to family therapist Wahida Chishti Valianti, in the article

"Challenges facing Muslim Families in North America" on the Web site *Islam, the Modern Religion* (February 2004).

See also: Divorce in America; Racially and Culturally Mixed Marriages

FURTHER READING
Netter, Perry. *Divorce Is a Mitzvah: A Practical Guide to Finding Wholeness and Holiness When Your Marriage Dies.* Woodstock, VT: Jewish Lights, 2002.
Jenks, Richard J. *Divorce, Annulments and the Catholic Church: Healing or Hurtful?* New York: Haworth, 2002.
Safi, Omid, ed. *Progressive Muslims: On Justice, Gender, and Pluralism.* Oxford: One World, 2003.

■ STEPFAMILIES
See: Children, Psychological Effects of Divorce on; Families, Blended

■ STRESS FACTORS IN MARRIAGE, EXTERNAL
The problems that arise through no fault of the husband or wife and that can harm a marriage.

In traditional wedding ceremonies, the bride and groom vow to remain together "for better, for worse, for richer, for poorer, in sickness and in health." The words are easily said but difficult to live up to.

Almost any long-term marriage will encounter a variety of external challenges that test the love, devotion, and toughness of each partner. Some events, such as a fire or the accidental death of a child, affect both partners equally. Others, such as job loss or the death of a parent, affect one more than the other, and the grieving or worried spouse turns to his or her partner for comfort and support.

These problems can put a strain on any marriage. In a troubled marriage, where the partners may have had difficulty relating to each other, a new stress can become the final blow that breaks up the marriage and leads to divorce.

DEATH IN A FAMILY
A young adult bride and groom may have the good fortune to see all four of their parents (and perhaps one or two stepparents) attend their wedding. At least some of this older generation may live close enough

to take on active grandparent roles when the couple has children. The married couple's siblings, living near or far, may become doting aunts and uncles, and, in many cases, friends, advisors, and confidants to the husband and/or wife.

When one of these close relatives dies, roles and routines may have to change to replace the "missing part" of the family. A serious illness among relatives can have a similar effect.

A grandparent or adult sibling with a degenerative disease (one that gets gradually more severe) such as Parkinson's or Alzheimer's, or who struggles with a **chronic illness** like heart disease or recurring cancers, can make enormous demands on a married couple. The ill person may require a major commitment of time, work, and sometimes money. The caregiving partner, most often the wife, can begin to feel she is cheating her own spouse or children of the attention they deserve, and her husband often agrees. If the situation lasts long enough, it can easily provoke conflict, just when sympathy and understanding are needed the most.

The death that often ensues can be devastating. The loss of a loved parent, especially one who played an active role in the adult child's life, often results in profound grief, guilt ("I could have done more"), resentment ("my spouse didn't let me do enough"), and self-pity. Childhood family dramas can be dredged up and mulled over in the weeks and months that follow. Bad feelings between the deceased and the son- or daughter-in-law, if not resolved before the death, can boil up again unexpectedly.

If the death of an aging parent can have such an effect, imagine how heartrending it must be for parents to lose a child to disease or accident. Such an event can pull a couple together—or push them apart. The bereaved parents probably feel the loss equally, unlike the situation with grandparents or adult siblings. However, different styles of grieving may mask their common grief and cause misunderstandings. Some couples benefit by joining one of the many support groups that now exist for grieving parents.

Fact Or Fiction?

Between 75 and 80 percent of married couples
divorce when one of their children dies.

Fact: No one knows the source of this widely cited myth, but it is not even remotely true. In 1999 a counseling group called Compassionate Friends surveyed 15,000 couples who suffered the loss of a child. Their overall divorce rate was not particularly high; furthermore, only 3 percent of the divorced couples believed that the death contributed to their divorce.

SERIOUS ILLNESS OR DISABILITY

Chronic illness or disability is not part of anyone's marriage plan. When it happens, it can upset all of a couple's dreams and expectations, throwing the marriage into question and even leading to divorce. After all, people get married to gain the support of a partner, not to acquire a lifelong patient.

When the sick partner is the family's breadwinner, the illness can result in a financial crisis—especially if there are medical or caretaking expenses not covered by health insurance. The healthy spouse may be forced to devote more hours to working outside the home, just when his or her services are in greatest demand *in* the home. The healthy spouse must nurse the sick one and take over his or her responsibilities with housework and child care.

Many chronically ill people lack the desire or ability to have sexual relations with their spouse, adding another level of frustration to the healthy spouse. In other cases, the healthy spouse may no longer feel attracted to a spouse who is ill or who has been in some way disfigured (had their appearance harmed) by disease or surgery.

Some chronic diseases can be fatal over the long term. The entire family may be living under that threat and an ongoing high level of stress and fear for the future.

Yet many families survive and thrive despite chronic illnesses. In an article in the journal *Peritoneal Dialysis International* in 1990, K.S. Lewis, whose own chronic illness brought an end to a 20-year marriage, discussed the "assets" that help many couples deal with the challenge: self-esteem; a long-lasting, previously happy marriage; similarity in age and religion; a helpful extended family; confidence about economic resources; and good friends.

The birth of a disabled or special needs child can also put pressure on a marriage. In addition to posing major demands on time, energy, and patience, the birth of a child with severe limitations is sometimes viewed as a blow to all the hopes and dreams of the parents. Feelings of guilt (however undeserved) and blame (however unfair) are fairly common in such situations.

According to divorce expert Judith Wallerstein in her 2000 book *The Unexpected Legacy of Divorce*, "Professional opinion [of psychologists] generally supports the clinical impression that divorce is higher" in families with special needs children, although no formal studies have been made to prove the connection.

TEENS SPEAK

Why Can't We All Be Happy?

Tanya was so happy three years ago when her mother gave birth to a baby boy. She had been an only child for 11 years, and now she had a brother. However, they soon realized that Joshie was severely disabled.

"I didn't care, because he was always so sweet. They let me hold him even when he still had the IV in his little neck. I love him so much, he laughs every time I go into his room and play with him, and he makes a lot of noises like talking. He likes my friends too, especially when we turn up the radio and dance."

Tanya's parents have spent a great deal of time, money, and physical effort to keep Joshie alive and healthy, though they still don't know whether he will ever be able to talk or walk by himself. But for the last year, their mother has been feeling the pressure.

"She goes away all the time to Lake Michigan by herself; sometimes she takes me too, but I don't want to go anymore. My Dad is so stubborn and he won't ever leave Joshie, but there's too much equipment to take over to the lake, and the nurse can't come either. Lately they have been fighting all the time. I think either Joshie goes to a home or they're going to get divorced. I'm very scared for all of us but I don't know what to do."

Tanya's parents have started counseling. She hopes they can work something out, because she loves both of them.

FINANCIAL DIFFICULTY

There is an old expression: "When poverty knocks at the door, love jumps out the window." You don't need to be rich to have a good marriage, but it certainly helps for a couple to have a steady, reliable income that covers the costs of feeding, clothing, entertaining, and educating children, and keeping them in good health. Childless couples feel economic pressures too, though perhaps not as critically.

Financial pressures are almost always present, even for middle-class families. People who are natural worriers have enough money worries to keep them occupied through decades of marriage. Even easygoing individuals may need to develop a thick skin in the face of all the unexpected expenses that are liable to hit any family.

Various studies and surveys over the years have consistently shown that couples with less money are more likely to have problems. People who are unable to support their families may lose their self-esteem.

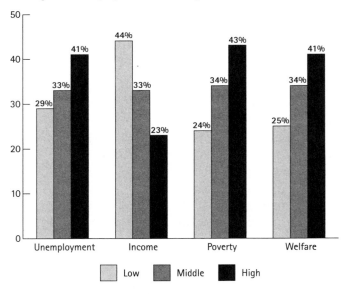

DID YOU KNOW?

Effect of Poverty on Divorce

Divorce rates are higher in communities with high unemployment, low income, and high rates of poverty and public assistance. The following table shows the percentage of divorce or separation in such communities. For example, neighborhoods with higher unemployment show higher rates of divorce.

Source: Centers for Disease Control and Prevention.

Unable to meet expectations, they may lash out in frustration at the first available target, their spouse or children. Accusations begin to multiply, such as "You're wasting my hard-earned money" or "You're not bringing in enough."

For example, a report published in 2002 in the journal *Demography* noted that according to several studies spanning the years 1950 to 1984, divorce rates were consistently higher for people with a lower economic status. The rates were higher despite the many social changes that took place during those years.

Couples can take steps to ease the pressure. Some set up weekly or monthly budgets to reduce the number of unpleasant surprises and to spread cutbacks evenly between the spouses; others meet with career counselors in public or private agencies, who may be able to help them exploit talents and skills they did not know they had; and still others learn, with the help of counselors, to avoid blaming each other for factors beyond their control, such as nationwide or local joblessness, or the high cost of living.

CAREER FAILURE, JOB LOSS, AND BUSINESS FAILURE

The loss of a job, the inability to get a promotion at work, or the failure of a small business can all strain a marriage. Apart from the money issues, these external crises can have devastating emotional effects on the person directly involved and on his or her spouse.

Success in business or the workplace has traditionally been a major factor in men's self-esteem. After the social changes of recent decades, many women also put great stock in holding the right job and securing the right promotion.

Workplace success translates to self-confidence in other areas as well and to a satisfying sense that one is able to support and even pamper his or her spouse and children. The reverse situation is also true. Someone who has lost a job, even through no fault of his or her own, often feels a sense of failure. Some withdraw emotionally from family members and even fall down on nonwork responsibilities.

The effects can be disastrous if the situation persists for long. According to divorce expert E. Mavis Hetherington, the rate of violence doubles in a family if the man is unemployed and the woman is working, though such responses are not typical. Well-adjusted people may be able to use downtime productively to build better ties with their children or to learn new work skills.

Q & A

Question: My dad just lost his job. Is there anything I can do to help out?

Answer: Not directly. He will have to find another job on his own. But you *can* be a little more reasonable about allowances and extra spending money until he does. Also, if you feel that he has the patience, you might suggest some activity you can do together that he didn't have the time to do when he was working, like going fishing or helping with a school project; just make sure it won't cost much money to do.

Most people like to believe that they value others based on their inner worth rather than their financial assets or success in the business world. Nevertheless, many men and women react badly to a decline in social status on the part of a spouse. In the past, women were often treated socially according to their husband's occupation. A job loss or business failure was a threat to the family's status and future, even to the children's marriage prospects.

Times have changed, but even today some spouses are apt to lose respect for a husband or wife who lacks or loses worldly success. These attitudes now apply to a degree to both sexes, as some men are attracted to women for their perceived success at work as much as for their nurturing abilities.

The timing of a job or business loss can be critical for a marriage too. A young person who is unemployed can probably find some other job before too long. Even when a particular business or industry goes out of style and a person's job skills become useless, younger people have the time and energy to build new careers. As people approach middle age, however, they usually find it harder to secure a new job in their old field, let alone in a new one. Middle-aged couples are often forced to reinvent their relationship as work and income patterns change. A fragile marriage can fall apart under this pressure.

MIDLIFE CRISIS

Sometimes age itself can put stress on a marriage, even those that have weathered two or three decades. The term **midlife crisis** was popularized in the 1970s by books like Gail Sheehy's best seller

Passages. It is still frequently used to describe the situation of people from about 39 through the mid-50s who experience anxieties about growing older and a new fear of death. Events like the birth of a grandchild or a sports injury may give a person a sudden unpleasant sense that he or she has aged before fulfilling long-held goals.

Typically, men are seen as more susceptible than women to midlife crises. On occasion, many people believe, the crisis can be severe enough to break up a marriage. However, a 2000 study published in the journal *Motivation and Emotion* reported that the incidence of midlife crisis has been exaggerated. Although a third of the hundreds of interviewed people between ages 40 and 53 claimed to have experienced a midlife crisis, more than half of them had merely been confronted by challenges common to any age group, which they successfully overcame. The study also found that women were as likely as men to go through midlife crises.

In any case, many people in the study used the crisis as an opportunity to find new meaning and direction in their lives. In other words, the latest research does not bear out the theory that midlife crisis is a significant threat to relationships.

Parents may ask kids to shoulder some of the added burden that external stresses place on their family. Older children should respond by showing understanding and cooperation, so as not to make a difficult situation even worse.

See also: Help for Troubled Marriages

FURTHER READING

American Cancer Society. *Couples Confronting Cancer: Keeping Your Relationship Strong.* Atlanta, GA: 2003.

McGonigle, Chris. *Surviving your Spouse's Chronic Illness.* New York: Henry Holt, 1999.

HOTLINES AND HELP SITES

A Kid's Guide to Divorce
URL: http://kidshealth.org/kid/feeling/home_family/divorce.html
Affiliation: Nemours Foundation's Center for Children's Health Media
Mission: To help kids understand the problems and issues they may
face when their parents divorce

Banana Splits: Children's Support Group
Phone: (212)262-4562
Mission: A school-based peer support program for children from
split families
Programs: Organizes support groups for children going through a
family divorce or experiencing problems due to divorce

Boys Town Hotline (for girls and boys)
Phone: 1-800-448-3000
Mission: To help children in any type of personal and family crisis
Programs: Trained counselors provide help for adults and kids dealing with abusive relationships, parent-child conflicts, pregnancy,
runaway youth, suicide, physical and sexual abuse. Operates 24
hours a day.

Connections for Children of Divorce
URL: http://www.geocities.com/Heartland/Shores/9064/Connectkids.
html
Mission: To provide resources and information regarding children
and divorce

Divorce Magazine

URL: http://www.divorcemag.com/indexCAN.shtml

Affiliation: consumer magazine

Mission: provides advice on every aspect of divorce, including the impact on children, with legal and other information for every U.S. state and Canadian province; has links to hundreds of local support groups

Kids Help Phone

URL: http://kidshelp.sympatico.ca/en/resources/sub_divorce.asp

Affiliation: Canadian nonprofit organization

Phone: 1-800-668-6868 (Canada)

Programs: Provides phone and online counseling; online forums to discuss divorce (and other topics); weekly chats on different topics; local chapters; student "ambassadors"

Kids Turn

URL: http://www.kidsturn.org/kids/aboutus.htm

Mission: To help younger children deal with parents' divorce

Programs: Provides information and fun activities

Stepfamily Association of America

URL: http://saafamilies.org/

Phone: 1-800-735-0329

Mission: Nonprofit membership organization dedicated to successful stepfamily living

Programs: Provides extensive online information about divorce and stepfamily living; online conferences for stepkids

GLOSSARY

adult children of divorce   a) adults whose parents divorced when they were young; or b) adult children of parents who **divorce**

adversarial   describes any process, like a criminal trial or a contested divorce, in which each side hires its own attorney and fights to protect its own interests, as opposed to reaching a voluntary compromise

alimony   lifelong monthly support payments from one divorced partner to the other; usually paid only to women who had been housewives in long-term marriages

annulment   a legal act that invalidates a marriage retroactively (after the fact) because, for example, one partner had misled the other; also used by the Roman Catholic and some other churches that do not recognize divorce

antimiscegenation laws   state laws in force prior to 1967 that made it a crime for people of different races to marry or to have sexual relations

anxiety   a feeling of worry, fear, and unease, often causing physical symptoms like sweating and heart palpitations

bankruptcy   a legal process that protects individuals (or businesses) who cannot pay their debts; usually, almost everything they own is divided among their creditors

battered woman syndrome   a psychological state in which a woman who has been abused by a partner loses the capacity or desire to resist abuse, or even denies that the abuse is taking place

bed and board divorce   a term used in a few states to describe a legal separation in which the marriage is not dissolved, but the court recognizes that the partners live apart and are not responsible for each other

behavior modification therapy   a form of therapy in which people learn to change the way they respond to a situation or problem

bigamy   having more than one husband or wife at the same time

birdnesting   a custody arrangement in which the children live in one residence all the time, and the divorced parents take turns living with them

caretaker   in the context of divorce, a child who takes on an adult role in family responsibilities, such as child care or chores

chronic illness   an illness that remains for a long period, or for life, and interferes with a person's normal functioning in life

civil union   a legal arrangement similar to marriage for same-sex couples

codependent   a person who devotes his or her life to a spouse or other individual (who may be addicted to alcohol or drugs), at the expense of the codependent's own life

cohabitation   living together as a couple without being married

collaborative divorce   a divorce in which the two partners try to negotiate their differences without going to court, with the help of lawyers who agree to be friendly rather than adversarial

common-law marriage   a legally recognized marriage in many states, in which two people have lived together as man and wife without a license for a certain number of years

community marriage policies (CMPs)   programs in which the clergy of various religious denominations in a town or city agree to perform marriage ceremonies only on couples who have been through pre-marital counseling and preparation

community property   all property that a married couple earned or obtained during their marriage plus any previous property that was jointly used by the couple; in the "community property states," this property is divided equally at the time of divorce

confidant   a person who shares intimate conversation and mutual advice with someone. Some children of divorce become a confidant to one parent.

co-parenting   an arrangement in which mother and father live in separate homes but share parenting responsibilities for their children. The parents can be married, divorced, or never married.

crude divorce rate   the number of divorces per 1,000 individuals of any age or sex

culture wars   political, legal, and intellectual conflicts between the more traditional and the more change-oriented groups in American society over social issues like marriage, child care, abortion, divorce, and homosexuality

custodial parent   the parent who has primary custody of the children after divorce

defendant   in divorce, the partner who did not file the divorce petition

deidealization   the process by which children gradually come to see their parents as real people, with strengths and weaknesses, needs and desires

depression   a psychological state marked by sadness, inactivity, inability to focus, and feelings of hopelessness

discovery   in divorce, the process of finding out exactly what financial assets each partner has; starts as soon as one partner files a divorce petition

divorce petition the legal paper a partner files with family court formally asking for a divorce

divorce settlement the legal agreement signed by divorcing partners and a family court judge, which tells exactly how to divide assets, how much support will be paid, if any, and how child custody will be divided

do-it-yourself divorce legal divorce obtained without the help of lawyers, or with minimum help

domestic partners two cohabiting people who have been recognized by an employer or a municipality as partners for the purpose of employee benefits, hospital visitation rights, etc.

domestic violence violence between family members

dowry the payment made by one party to a marriage (either the bride, the groom, or one of their families) to the other party

dysfunctional family a family in which the parents are unable or unwilling to carry out their responsibilities and lack normal caring relationships

emotional distance a lack of interest in a partner's emotional needs and desires

enabling the practice of cooperating with addicted loved ones in their addictive behavior

equitable distribution a fair distribution of assets that takes into account non-financial contributions to a marriage and family; formerly the division of assets after a divorce based on whose name was on the property deeds or accounts

family support programs programs run by government or private agencies to provide counseling as well as practical support in helping to keep families together

fault divorce   a divorce in which one party formally accuses the other of misconduct

five stages of grief   the emotional phases people often go through when they confront death or any other serious loss, such as the breakup of a family

fixed visitation schedule   a custody-sharing arrangement in which each parent's time with the children is provided for exactly in the settlement

gay   a common term for **homosexual**

goodwill   in the sale or division of a business or a professional practice, an asset that represents the business's reputation and stable customer base. It may be included in calculating division of assets in a divorce

gray divorce   divorce of partners in a long-term marriage who have reached middle age

half-sibling   a brother or sister who has the same biological mother but different biological father—or vice versa

heterosexual   being emotionally and sexually attracted to people of the opposite sex

hidden agendas   issues that people may *really* be concerned about, though they don't actually bring them up in a discussion or argument

homosexual   being emotionally and sexually attracted to people of one's own sex

intercultural couple   a couple from ethnically or religiously different backgrounds

interfaith marriage   a marriage between people of different religions

interreligious couple   a couple from different religious backgrounds

intimate partner violence (IPV) domestic violence between two people who are married, cohabiting, or dating

joint legal custody a child custody arrangement following divorce in which both parents have the right to participate in decisions about their children's health, education, and way of life

joint physical custody a child custody arrangement following divorce in which the children live at least 30 percent of the time with each parent

legal custody the power to make binding decisions about a couple's children, including health, education, and way of life, such as the school they will attend and the religion they will practice

legal separation a legally recognized status in which a married couple agree to live apart without getting divorced

litigation a legal proceeding in court, usually pursued in an **adversarial** manner

living wills a document instructing doctors and hospitals as to a patient's wishes should they become incapacitated; it may designate a spouse or other person as executor

longitudinal study a medical or sociological study that follows a group over a period of many years in order to see the long-term effects of inputs like medicines, diets, or divorce

mediation in divorce, a method in which the partners work out a settlement voluntarily with the help of professionals, but avoiding litigation

midlife crisis a situation in which a middle aged individual becomes emotionally unstable due to fears about getting old

monogamy having only one partner at a time

no-fault divorce divorce granted to either spouse without having to prove misconduct by the other spouse

noncustodial parent   after a divorce or separation, the parent who has custody of the children for a good deal less than half the time, if at all, and/or who has no legal control over decisions affecting the children's lives

nuclear family   a family composed of father, mother, and their biological children

open marriage   A marriage in which the partners allow each other to have intimate relations and affairs with other people

open relationship   a relationship of any kind in which the partners allow each other to have intimate relations or affairs with other people

overburdened children   children of divorce who assume many adult responsibilities due to inadequate parenting by the custodial parent

permanent support   spousal support payments required by the divorce settlement. These payments are usually not for life and are "permanent" only in comparison to the temporary support during predivorce separation.

physical custody   the parent with whom the children live

plaintiff   in divorce law, the person who files the divorce petition

polygamy   having two or more spouses at the same time

POSSLQ   an acronym used by the Census Bureau for "persons of the opposite sex sharing living quarters." The assumption is that most of these people are cohabiting couples.

power of attorney   the power granted in a will or other legal document to carry out the intentions of the person who drew up the document

prenuptial agreement   a legal contract drawn up between two people before they marry, specifying how property and income will be shared during the marriage and, most importantly, after a divorce

primary caretaker   the person who did most of the care of the children while the marriage was intact

primary custodial parent   the parent who has physical custody of the children most of the time

protection order   a legal document issued by a judge ordering someone to stay away from another person or family; it is issued when there is valid reason to fear violence or abuse

rape   forcing another person (usually a woman) to have sex against his or her will through violence or threats; having sex with a person who is too young or too incapacitated to consent

reasonable visitation   a visitation plan in some divorce settlements that doesn't specify exactly how much time the noncustodial parent has with the children

refined divorce rate   the number of divorces per 1,000 married women

replacement value   the cost of replacing an asset (such as a car, or a piece of furniture) by buying a new one

respondent   the person who is called upon to respond to a divorce petition; usually the spouse of the person filing the petition

response   the reply that the respondent makes to the statements in the divorce petition

separate maintenance   another term for **bed and board divorce**

serial monogamy   The practice of being married and divorced several times, while remaining faithful to each partner while the marriage lasts

shared custody   legal or physical custody that is divided between two parents at least to some degree

significant other   a general term to refer to someone's partner, whether married, live-in, or dating exclusively

sole physical custody an arrangement in which the children live with one parent all the time

split physical custody an arrangement in which children are divided between the two parents, at least part of the time

spousal maintenance court-ordered payments from one partner to another after divorce, only for a limited period while the recipient learns job skills

stepsibling a brother or sister with different biological parents who live in the same family, due to divorce (or death) and remarriage

straight heterosexual

supervised visits visits between a parent and children in the presence of a neutral adult; visits are supervised when there is legitimate fear of violence or abuse

temporary support court-ordered support payments from one spouse to another during legal separation but before divorce

tender years doctrine the idea, now rejected by most people, that children should always live with their mother after divorce, at least if they are under 8 years old

trial separation a period of time during which a married couple lives apart, while they consider whether or not they want to save their marriage

visitation rights the court-ordered rights of the noncustodial parent to have the children stay at his home for limited periods of time, or to visit with the children at a neutral place

INDEX

Page numbers in *italic* indicate graphs or sidebars. Page numbers in **bold** denote main entries.